EATING FOR A
HEALTHY
HEART

Explaining the 'French Paradox'

Professor John S Yudkin and Sara Stanner

D1323997

BBC BOOKS

ACKNOWLEDGEMENTS

We are grateful to Professor Walter Willett, Coordinator of the Nurses' Health Study, and Professor Serge Renaud, father of the French Paradox, for encouragement and comments on our book. We also thank Professor Tom Sanders for the use of his food analysis programme and Angela Ryle, Senior Dietician at the Whittington Hospital, London, for her help and advice.

Proceeds from this book will be used to fund research in the Centre for Diabetes and Cardiovascular Risk of UCL Medical School at the Whittington Hospital, and we would like to thank Delia Smith, Sophie Grigson, Valentina Harris, Mireille Johnston and Claudia Roden for their generosity and use of their recipes.

Published by BBC Books,
an imprint of BBC Worldwide Publishing.
BBC Worldwide Limited, Woodlands,
80 Wood Lane, London W12 0TT

First published 1996
text © Professor John S Yudkin and Sara Stanner 1996
wine text © Malcolm Gluck
recipes © Sophie Grigson, Valentina Harris, Mireille Johnston,
Claudia Roden and Delia Smith
The moral rights of the authors have been asserted

ISBN 0 563 37165 X

Photographs by Professor John S Yudkin
except page 21 © 1995 MC Escher/Cordon Art, Baarn, Holland
(all rights reserved) and page 80 © 1995 Richard Jenkins
Recipe photographs by Alex Dufort, Graham Kirk, Peter Knab, Jess Koppel, James Murphy,
Simon Smith at Barry Bullough Studios and Grant Symons © BBC Books
Illustrations by Sweeta Patel

Designed and set by BBC Books
Set in A Garamond
Colour origination by Radstock Reproductions Ltd, Midsomer Norton
Printed by Cambus Litho Ltd, East Kilbride
Bound by Hunter and Foulis Ltd, Edinburgh
Cover printed by Clays Ltd, St Ives plc

Contents

Professor John S. Yudkin MD FRCP

John S. Yudkin is Professor of Medicine at University College London, and works as a consultant in General Medicine and Diabetes at the Whittington Hospital in north London. His department is involved in a busy research programme on the causes and prevention of heart disease in people both with and without diabetes. He has strong family connections with an interest in diet and heart disease: his uncle, Professor John Yudkin, who died in 1995, wrote extensively about sugar and health.

Ms Sara Stanner BSc

Sara Stanner is a research administrator in the Department of Medicine, University College London Medical School. She is currently coordinating a project in the Former Soviet Union to look at the effects of intra-uterine starvation, during the siege of Leningrad, on adult diabetes and heart disease.

FOREWORD

This is a very special book about a subject on which a zillion books have already been written. But what makes this one different is that it is written by two people who are eminently qualified to write on the subject – a doctor (John S. Yudkin) and a nutritionist (Sara Stanner). John Yudkin is a highly respected Professor of Medicine at University College London, and he is a passionate lover of good food and wine. His experience of the tragic loss of his own father from a heart attack at a very early age will, I know, have added a deeply personal edge to his research into the high incidence of such premature deaths in Britain.

John is also a personal friend and I cut my teeth in cooking, as it were, preparing meals for his delightful family way back in the sixties when he was still a young medical student. Since then we continue to share animated discussions on recipes and cooking, and our passion for our respective football teams.

In unravelling the French Paradox, John Yudkin and his coauthor Sara Stanner present a very positive vision of healthy eating. Too often I feel healthy regimes are presented to us as strict puritanical messages which makes them hard to stick to. Here, instead of the killjoy message we are used to, we find that medical knowledge and the best in modern cookery writing can be combined to get the right balance so that everyone can enjoy a good diet and good health at the same time.

Delia Smith

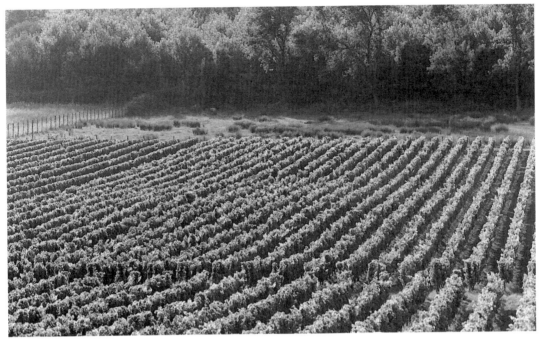

The vineyards of Bordeaux produce some of the most elegant and expensive red wines in the world and, as we will explain, these may be good for your heart as well as your soul!

INTRODUCTION

'These are old fond paradoxes to make fools laugh i' the alehouse.'

OTHELLO, ACT 2, SCENE 1; SHAKESPEARE

Oh no! Not another book about dieting! More advice about how we can live longer, stay healthier, or lose 12 pounds in a fortnight. Another set of 'experts' with some new set of ideas which disagree with everything that the last lot of 'experts' told us. What's bad for us now? What's the next thing we have to give up that we really enjoy?

A very understandable reaction! Every few months newspapers have another article about scientific studies which show that this or that is good, or bad, for you. And we get panels of experts telling us what we must cut down on, and how many potatoes or slices of bread we should be eating each day. More often than not, we are told that the things which are bad for us are the ones we really enjoy, and what we *should* be eating are the things that aren't much fun. Why is it that we're reminded of those days in short trousers or pigtails, being told to 'eat your greens/spinach/carrots because they're good for you' or 'if you carry on eating crisps or chocolate/drinking lemonade you will get really fat/lose your teeth/never get rid of those spots'?

Perhaps it's because food experts are constantly telling us what we should eat, and shouldn't eat, rather than putting more emphasis on what is fun and healthy to eat. Food should be enjoyable.

People derive pleasure from eating good, wholesome food and from sharing meals. There's no such thing as 'good' or 'bad' foods. It's what we eat and drink overall that's important. And it's variety that creates a 'balanced diet' and makes eating more enjoyable. A Big Mac with cheese, for example, or a chocolate éclair, is not going to do you any harm – as long as that's not what you eat, and all you eat, day in and day out.

What's different, then, about this book? Just a new set of experts with a new lot of do's and don'ts? We don't think so. This is a book about a paradox – defined in our dictionaries as a puzzle or a contradiction. The paradox is that, as a nation, the French have a risk of heart attacks which is only around one-quarter or one-third of that in the United Kingdom. And this is despite the fact that, by most of the measures used to judge heart attack risk, the French should be much higher on the heart attack league table. Even within France there is a gradient of heart attack rates, with people in the south less at risk than those from further north. And in this regard, the Mediterranean French share their low rates of heart disease with other countries around the Mediterranean, suggesting that what we should be looking for to explain the French Paradox is not just a French phenomenon. But in France, the paradox is most apparent: a Western European lifestyle, what seem to be high levels of risk, but low rates of heart disease.

The search for the explanation to this paradox has focused on what the French eat and drink. So, if the French really do suffer fewer heart attacks than would be expected from their cholesterol levels, their blood pressure and their smoking habits, is it because they are denying themselves the pleasures of food? We hardly think so! If any nation ever justified a reputation for making the preparation, consumption and enjoyment of food into a religion, it is France. So there may be something about what the French eat (not forgetting what they drink) that will make it necessary to rethink some of our old views on the causes of heart attacks. And that's what this book is about.

The French Paradox is a book about enjoying food and drink and staying healthy. It gets away from the idea that a diet must all be about what *not* to eat and what to cut out. This book is designed as a recipe to get you thinking about food and drink and health in a different, and positive way. It's a mixture of theory and practice, in three sections:

• a section outlining the ideas of the French Paradox;
• a section on the choice of red wines available;
• and a section of recipes based on the concepts introduced in the first section.

In the first part, we'll set out the facts and figures which have led to the idea of the French Paradox. We will explain what we mean by heart attacks and atherosclerosis (there is a glossary on page 156 to help explain some of the medical or scientific terms we use), and look at some of the problems of the traditional 'cholesterol = heart attack' view as to what causes heart disease. We'll then outline several

of the candidates which might explain the French Paradox. In so doing, we'll discuss some of the new ideas about atherosclerosis and heart attacks which make the French Paradox less of a puzzle. These new insights recognize:

• that it is not just the level of cholesterol that matters, but its nature;
• that other things, such as blood clotting, alter the risk of heart attacks;
• and that what we eat and drink can have major effects on all these things.

Above all, the example which the French set the British and many other nations is how to enjoy food and wine. For this reason we're not producing just a textbook of theory about heart attacks.

The second section is all about wine. At first sight, this might seem quite surprising in a book which is supposed to be about health. But as you'll see, we aim to persuade you that part of the explanation of the French Paradox might be something to do with what's in a glass of wine. And that a person who drinks a couple of glasses of wine a day is less likely to get a heart attack than either a teetotaller or a spirit or beer drinker. It's for this reason that we use this section of the book to try to help you with choosing, buying and appreciating wine to match your meals.

In the last section we have put together some 50 different recipes from five of the best known cooks in Britain. And these put the emphasis on enjoying cooking and eating, using ingredients and cooking styles which have a predominantly Mediterranean flavour.

At the end, you'll find a glossary of terms to help you understand some of the technical jargon, although you'll be quite familiar with the vocabulary very soon.

Settle down, tuck in your napkin, and enjoy!

1

CORONARY HEART DISEASE – WHAT AND WHY?

'… how ill all's here about my heart.'
HAMLET, ACT 5, SCENE 2; SHAKESPEARE

In this chapter we will explain some of the terms that we'll use throughout this book. We will explain what we mean by a heart attack, by atherosclerosis and by coronary heart disease, and we'll make connections with similar diseases in other parts of the body. We will talk about why coronary heart disease is so important, both for doctors and for the general public. We will then go on to look at what happens to the heart and its blood supply when things go wrong, in order to tackle the important question: what causes coronary heart disease?

We believe that if we ask each of you, our readers, that same question, a lot of you would already have fairly strong views. We'd probably get lots of answers like 'cholesterol', 'a bad diet' and 'stress', with some other replies thrown into the melting pot, such as 'smoking' and 'taking no exercise'. For this very reason – that there are lots of conceptions, and misconceptions, about the cause of heart disease – we'll also spend some time tackling some of these myths.

WHAT IS CORONARY HEART DISEASE?

The heart is a lump of muscle weighing about 340 grams, or three-quarters of a pound. Its job is to act as a very powerful pump. It has two pairs of chambers, two right-sided and two left. The right half pumps blood through the lungs to pick up oxygen, while the left pumps this oxygen-rich blood through the rest of the body. It has to beat 60 or 70 times a minute, and more if we do anything energetic, from long-before-cradle to grave. If you work it out, this means that the average heart beats around 3,000,000,000 times in its lifetime.

Because it has so much work to do, just like any machine, the heart needs a lot of fuel and oxygen for energy, and it gets these from its own blood supply. And because it's beating day and night without stopping, the heart uses up around 20 per cent of the total oxygen intake in order to convert its fuel supply into energy. The blood vessels which supply the heart are called coronary arteries. There are two

The human heart

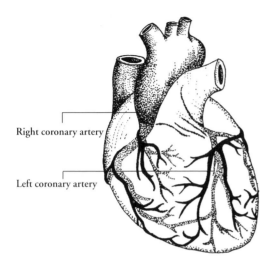

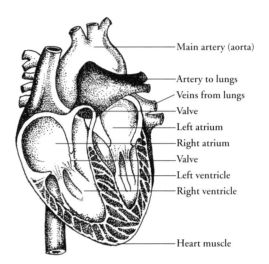

Main artery (aorta)
Artery to lungs
Veins from lungs
Valve
Left atrium
Right atrium
Valve
Left ventricle
Right ventricle
Heart muscle

Right coronary artery

Left coronary artery

of these, the right and the left, but the latter in turn divides into two large branches (see above).

Coronary heart disease (or coronary artery disease) is what happens when these blood vessels become narrowed or blocked. The narrowing process is the result of changes in the wall of the coronary arteries called atherosclerosis or arteriosclerosis. The wall of the artery is invaded by cells which become loaded with a fatty substance called cholesterol. Our body needs this cholesterol, because in health it's used to build up the walls surrounding each cell. But in disease, when the number of these cholesterol-loaded cells builds up, they produce frothy-looking cells filled with cholesterol and other fats. These are called foam cells (see right).

Some of these eventually die and release their cholesterol content. And this in turn leads to a large collection of this fatty material in the wall of the artery. This is known as an atherosclerotic plaque. Whereas healthy arteries are springy or elastic, atherosclerotic plaques are stiff and may crack. The stiffness of atherosclerotic plaques is why people talk about hardening of the arteries.

Formation of foam cells leading to heart disease

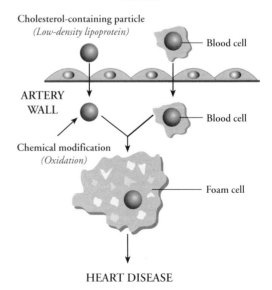

BLOOD

Cholesterol-containing particle
(Low-density lipoprotein)

Blood cell

ARTERY WALL

Blood cell

Chemical modification
(Oxidation)

Foam cell

HEART DISEASE

CROSS-SECTION OF AN ARTERY PARTIALLY OBSTRUCTED BY AN ATHEROSCLEROTIC PLAQUE

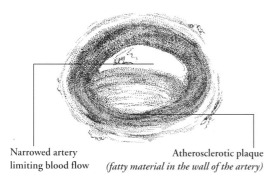

Narrowed artery
limiting blood flow

Atherosclerotic plaque
(fatty material in the wall of the artery)

These atherosclerotic plaques can produce damage in one of two ways. Firstly, by their very size, they cause narrowing of the artery. This limits the amount of blood that can be pumped through to feed the heart. The heart uses more fuel and more oxygen when it's pumping more forcefully, or more quickly, so narrowed arteries are more likely to cause problems when someone exercises. The result is that people feel a cramping pain across their chest, which usually starts when they exert themselves and passes off within a few minutes when they stop. This is known as angina.

The second thing that can happen is that an atherosclerotic plaque acts as the focus for a blood clot or thrombosis. Although this can happen to the plaque at any time, we think that it's more likely to happen if the plaque ruptures, or cracks. A normal blood vessel does not allow blood to clot inside it, mainly because the lining cells have a very powerful ability to block the clotting process. But if a plaque bursts, blood gets into the inside of the artery wall where all the cholesterol has accumulated. So the blood finds itself free of the anti-clotting properties of the lining cells. And something else that's increasingly obvious is that the risk of a heart attack is higher in people whose blood is more likely to clot. This may be because the cells which start the clotting process, the platelets, are more sticky.

Or it can happen when there are high levels of certain blood-clotting chemicals in the blood. If so, the blood may stick to the blood vessel wall where it's rough and irregular over an atherosclerotic plaque, even without the plaque cracking.

When a clot occurs in a coronary artery, the result is a heart attack or myocardial infarction. These words literally translate as 'death of the heart muscle as a result of cutting off its blood supply'. A person who suffers a myocardial infarction usually feels severe pain across the chest, perhaps going down into the left arm or up to the neck, and they may sweat and feel sick and breathless. Unlike with angina, the pain usually starts without any exercise, and is not relieved by sitting or lying still, or by taking pills or medicine that usually help angina. A heart attack is a medical emergency, but with modern treatment, including the use of 'clot-busting' drugs, somewhere around 85-90 per cent of people taken to hospital with a heart attack now survive.

Heart failure is a term that doctors use to mean that the heart is not pumping as well as it should. The usual result is that fluid builds up – either in the lungs (which causes breathlessness during exercise, or when someone lies down) or in the legs. The commonest cause of heart failure is coronary artery disease. Surprisingly, many people who suffer heart failure caused by coronary artery disease have never noticed any chest pain, either from angina or from a heart attack.

The process of atherosclerosis is not limited to the arteries of the heart. Most arteries in the body can be affected. Apart from the coronary arteries, the blood vessels most commonly involved are those to the brain and the legs. A thrombosis, or blood clot in an artery supplying the brain, will produce a stroke, usually causing paralysis of part of the body. If the arteries to the legs are narrowed, this can produce painful cramp in the muscles of the calf or thigh during exercise; this is called claudication. A blood clot, or thrombus, in this artery might cause the death of the tissues of the toes or feet, known as gangrene.

Having explained what we mean by the terms we use, let's go on to give some facts and figures.

CORONARY HEART DISEASE – A MAJOR CAUSE OF ILL HEALTH

Coronary heart disease is a major killer in most countries of the industrialized world. In the UK, statistics show that just over one person in four dies of a heart attack, or from heart failure caused by coronary heart disease (see right). If one adds to this the number of deaths and the number of people disabled through suffering strokes, and from damage to arteries in other parts of the body, well over one-third of all deaths are a result of atherosclerosis.

We have said that coronary heart disease is a problem throughout the industrialized world, but the situation in the UK is an extreme cause for concern. When the league tables are drawn up for deaths from coronary heart disease (see below), Scotland is now the undoubted champion, with

CAUSES OF DEATH IN THE UK IN 1992

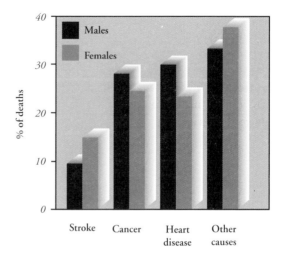

Ireland, England and Wales not far behind. This is not a league championship to be proud of.

Several other countries which were once very high on the list have now dropped their heart attack risk substantially. In particular, the death

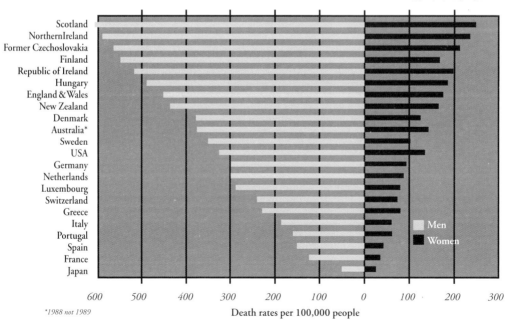

DEATH RATES FROM HEART DISEASE IN MEN AND WOMEN AGED 35–74 (1989)

Death rates per 100,000 people

*1988 not 1989

rate from coronary heart disease in the United States has fallen by around one half in the last fifteen years.

But when we look at other parts of the world, we find some countries where heart attack rates are extremely low. Death rates from heart disease in Japan are only around one-tenth of those in the UK. And in many parts of Africa, any form of atherosclerosis is rare.

VARIATIONS IN CORONARY HEART DISEASE – CLUES ABOUT THE CAUSES

What causes such large differences in rates of disease in different populations and countries (see graphs below)? Does this provide clues to what causes, and hints as to how to prevent, coronary heart disease?

The first possible explanation for differences in

DEATH RATES FROM HEART DISEASE IN MEN AGED 35–74 (1968–91)

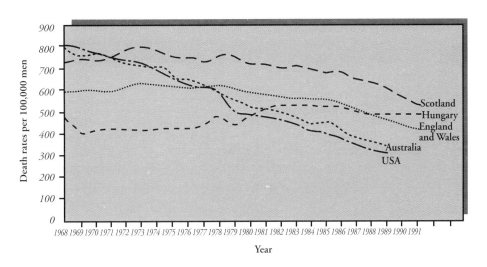

DEATH RATES FROM HEART DISEASE IN WOMEN AGED 35–74 (1968–91)

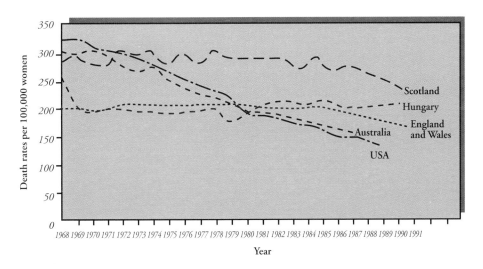

heart attack rates between countries is that it's all to do with heredity. Are there genes that protect us from heart disease, with some populations, or some individuals, being more at risk than others? It's certainly true that heart disease runs in families, especially if it develops at a young age. But there's really no likelihood that differences in heart disease rates between countries has much to do with inheritance. This is most obvious when we look at people who move from one country to another. In the early part of the twentieth century, large numbers of people emigrated from Japan to Hawaii, and then on to the west coast of the United States. Within two generations, the heart attack rates among these Japanese Americans were as high as those in Americans of European origin. And what this represented was around a six-fold increase in coronary heart disease risk within two generations.

IF IT'S NOT OUR GENES, THEN WHAT IS IT?

The science of epidemiology is gowing in importance. It is the study of patterns of disease, occurring both within and between populations.

Epidemiologists study the particular characteristics of people who already have a disease and compare them with people who haven't. More importantly, epidemiologists look at large numbers of people who are healthy, take all sorts of measurements, and then wait to see who does become ill. In other words, these studies will tell us which of a person's characteristics make a disease more likely to develop in the future.

This is important, because if certain factors differ between people with a disease and people without a disease, it's not clear which is the cause and which is the effect. For example, we might find that levels of certain vitamins in the blood are lower in people who have a stomach ulcer. But whether the low vitamin level causes the ulcer, or the ulcer lowers the vitamin level, can't be answered. So we need to find out whether healthy people with low levels of the vitamin are more likely to develop an ulcer.

The characteristics of a person and their lifestyle which enable us to predict illness are known as risk factors. If you ask anyone to name three risk factors for coronary heart disease you can be sure that cholesterol will be on every list. And it's certainly true that a measurement of the level of cholesterol in the blood gives some indication of that person's risk of getting, or dying from, coronary heart disease. Cholesterol is measured in millimoles per litre, usually abbreviated to mmol per litre. In Britain, the average cholesterol level is around 6 mmol per litre. For someone with a level of over 7 mmol per litre, the heart attack risk is increased by around 50 per cent compared to people with levels of 6. If, however, the level is under 5 mmol per litre, the risk of coronary heart disease is around 40 per cent lower.

ESTIMATED RISE IN DEATHS FROM CORONARY HEART DISEASE IN MEN IN THE UK AND USA AT EACH LEVEL OF CHOLESTEROL CONCENTRATION

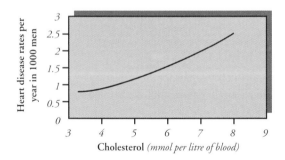

Let's move on, in our opinion poll, to ask what causes people to have a high or a low cholesterol level. The majority view would relate it to how much butter and cheese, cream and fatty meat the person eats. This has led to a straight line view of the connection:

Animal fat ➤ Blood cholesterol ➤ Heart attacks

This is a model which is commonly called the 'Diet-heart Model' of heart disease. And it's our starting point in talking about healthy eating. But what we're going to do is to use it as an Aunt Sally: to set it up in order to knock it down again.

As is the case for many old and long-established beliefs, there's certainly a grain of truth in this model. But what we're concerned about is how little can be explained by such a simple view of heart disease.

So what have we got against this traditional view? There are a number of factors to consider.

CHOLESTEROL IN THE BLOOD

To start with, the level of cholesterol in the blood is influenced by a whole range of things. Only one of these is the amount of fatty meat and dairy products we eat. It's certainly true that some of the differences between countries in the average cholesterol levels is partly explained by the diet people eat. In Japan or China, for example, where animal fats make up a much smaller proportion of the diet, the average cholesterol level is around 4 mmol per litre, compared with 6 mmol per litre in the UK.

But when we look for connections between cholesterol levels and people's diet within a population, these links are very weak. The explanation for this is not clear. It may be that it's not one's present diet that affects cholesterol levels, but one's diet over many years. And perhaps it is also that, like the Japanese, we need to cut out most of the animal fat in our diet to make any sizeable effect on these levels.

DIETARY CHANGES

When people make small changes to their diet, the impact on cholesterol levels is fairly small. Cutting visible fat off meat, using semi-skimmed milk, and putting only a thin spreading of butter on bread will lower the cholesterol level by only around 5 per cent. More extreme diets, such as vegan diets, lower cholesterol rather more, but many people would not enjoy them and extreme diets may cause other medical problems.

What about the cholesterol itself in the diet? Diets which are rich in animal fat also contain a lot of cholesterol. Other foods, such as eggs, are also rich in cholesterol without being thought of as traditionally 'fatty' foods. The amount of cholesterol in the diet affects cholesterol levels, but only to a fairly small degree. So here, again, we can't blame heart disease on eating too much cholesterol.

Both these points make it clear that we need to adapt the Diet-heart Model we drew on page 14. High cholesterol levels may be bad for your heart, but that's not just the result of cream cakes. But, this is not saying that animal fat is good for your heart. It may do harm in lots of other ways, as we'll soon see.

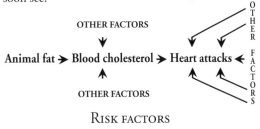

RISK FACTORS

Our next point is that cholesterol is only one of several factors which increase the risk of coronary heart disease – and not even the most important one. We have outlined above what we mean by risk factors – the characteristics of a person which increase their risk of getting heart disease. Apart from cholesterol, there are two other main risk factors which affect large numbers of people, and which we ourselves can influence. These are high blood pressure and smoking.

But if you thought that the list stopped there unfortunately it's not as simple as that. At the last count, more than 300 risk factors for coronary heart disease had been published in different scientific studies. This certainly weakens the claim of the old, rather simplified, Diet-heart Model!

Even in comparison with our two other main risk factors, blood pressure and smoking, cholesterol is fairly weak. We have calculated that, for a 45-year-old man, having a high cholesterol level (which we've defined as being in the top 20 per cent of the population) shortens one's life by 2½ years compared to that for someone with a lower level. If, however, that man's blood pressure were in the top 20 per cent, his life expectancy would be shortened by 5½ years. And if he smoked, he'd be estimated to shorten his life expectancy by 7½ years. So cholesterol is not only one risk factor among many, it's not even the most important.

EFFECT OF RISK FACTORS FOR HEART DISEASE ON THE LIFE EXPECTANCY OF A 45-YEAR-OLD MAN IN UK

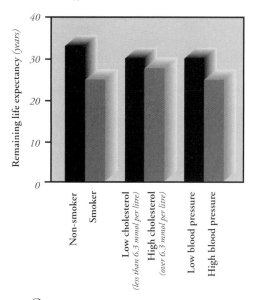

OTHER EFFECTS OF A HIGH-FAT DIET

The next point about the Diet-heart Model is that fatty meat and dairy products may do harmful things besides affecting the cholesterol level. Looking down the list of risk factors, several different characteristics of the blood, besides cholesterol levels, in turn increase the risk of atherosclerosis or of blood clotting (thrombosis). And some of these can be affected by animal fat intake, regardless of what happens to cholesterol.

The danger of the Diet-heart Model is the assumption that anything that affects the heart is

channelled through cholesterol. And this idea would almost give free licence to eat as much animal fat as we like as long as one's cholesterol is okay. This is clearly not the case.

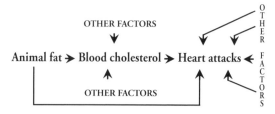

PREVENTION OF HEART DISEASE

What we think is by far and away the most serious problem about the Diet-heart Model is what it produces in the way of implications for preventing heart disease. For a long time now, health education about heart disease has advocated reducing the intake of animal fats, and substituting these with polyunsaturates from vegetable oils, in spreads and for cooking.

Replacing some of the animal fat in the diet with vegetable oils does have an effect on lowering cholesterol levels, even if it's not as big as one might hope. And it's this observation which has led to our traditional views about eating for a healthy heart. The message has been to replace butter, lard and dripping with margarine and cooking oil. And over the last generation, the rise in coronary heart disease rates, which was such a cause for concern in the 1970s, has flattened off and, in many countries, actually fallen. Isn't this proof, then, that the Diet-heart Model is right? And that polyunsaturates are good for you?

We think not, and for two reasons. The first is that in the United States, where the drop in heart disease rates has been the most marked, this fall has been similar in men and women, skilled and unskilled, young and old, black and white – not all of whom have changed their diet and lifestyle to the same degree. This would suggest a general trend, not obviously linked to changes in lifestyle.

But there is a second point, and perhaps the

more important one. It is that two studies have actually looked at coronary heart disease rates in people who have filled in detailed dietary surveys to see how much animal fat and margarine they eat. One was conducted with some 121,700 nurses in America, and the other in about 2500 men in Wales. And in both studies, those people eating the most margarine had the highest rates of heart attacks. The changes in the processing of oils to make soft margarine, which have largely taken over the market in the last fifteen years, just make it possible that these findings could be irrelevant today. We'll be returning to this whole question in Chapter 3. But let's just make the point here that cutting animal fat by substituting with polyunsaturates may not be as simple an answer as we thought; or it may not even be any answer.

RETHINKING THE DIET-HEART MODEL

This book is an attempt to reprogramme your thinking on the link between your diet and your heart. We think that there *is* a strong connection. But we think that cholesterol, at least in its old role, is not at the centre of the argument. There are lots of things which affect the development of atherosclerosis which have nothing to do with cholesterol.

Modern science has delved and probed and put together some fascinating new insights into how these risk factors operate. This has led to a new model linking diet to heart disease. The next few chapters will outline the growing agreement about the causes of coronary heart disease, and will point out, among other things:

• that it's not just the level of cholesterol which matters but its chemical nature;

• to suffer from a heart attack you don't just need atherosclerosis in your coronary artery, but a blood clot, or thrombosis, as well. Several risk factors, or protective factors, may operate through this blood clotting mechanism rather than through atherosclerosis.

But before we go on to outline some of these new ideas, let's say a few words about the different sorts of scientific studies we'll be throwing at you, the nature of the evidence. Why is it that we get such conflicting advice from experts? New research studies give us constantly changing views about what different things in the diet do. And as a result, the experts seem to differ in what they consider to be a healthy diet. We used to be told that 'stodgy' foods, such as bread and potatoes, were fattening and so they were bad for us. But now the experts seem to agree that we should be eating more, and not less, starchy carbohydrates. So why the conflict of evidence?

There are several different reasons for this. The results of a research study will depend on the question that the study is asking, and how it is being asked. The population being studied may be different, or the preparation, or food, being tested may also differ. And the thing that is being measured may also make the difference between a 'positive' and a 'negative' result. What we should be interested in is heart attack rates. But if you want to do a study showing that a particular food affects this risk, you'd need to look at several thousand people, and you'd have to follow them up over perhaps five or ten years. What's more, the only 100 per cent convincing way to do the trial is by giving two identical groups of people a diet which was exactly the same with the sole exception of the food under study. And even if this were possible, or ethical, it would still take a very long time to discover anything at all.

This is why many studies don't use what the epidemiologists call 'hard end-points', like heart attacks or deaths. They use instead a substitute, or surrogate, end-point. And the most common surrogate end-point in studies of this nature is the blood cholesterol level! If one really believes that cholesterol is right at the centre of the whole cause of coronary heart disease, then it's fine as a surrogate. But we've already challenged this idea. What this means is that something may well affect the level of cholesterol in a good direction, but may have a less good, or even harmful, effect on heart attack risk.

There's one way around the problem of large intervention studies and of surrogate end-points. And this is to compare patterns of disease in different countries with very different diets. About thirty years ago, Ancel Keys, an American epidemiologist, looked at rates of heart attacks in seven countries around the world. He showed that people in the United States were five or six times more likely to die from heart attacks than people in Greece.

INCIDENCE OF HEART DISEASE IN MEN IN THE SEVEN COUNTRIES STUDY UNDERTAKEN IN THE 1960S

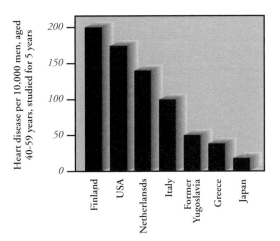

Since then there have been many other studies comparing national rates of heart disease and how they relate to differences in diet. And these studies can show that very different diets and different disease rates seem to go hand in hand. But there's always the problem – that people in Heraklion, Greece, will differ from people in High Wycombe, England, in many more ways than in what they eat. We will be coming back to some of these studies later on.

An enormous amount of very valuable information can come from studies of diet and disease *within* populations. Perhaps the most remarkable of all such studies is the Nurses' Health Study in the United States, which we've already mentioned in passing. This began in 1976 when 121,700 nurses completed questionnaires about their usual diet, and gave details of their medical history. Over the last two decades, it's been possible to relate different things that these nurses reported that they ate to a higher or lower risk of getting a whole range of diseases. We'll also be coming back to this study several times.

A whole range of different markers, then, are used to support claims for different things in the diet. All these markers have advantages – even if it's just that it's a surrogate end-point to measure. So we are going to have to do what everybody else does: use a whole range of different types of study to support the arguments that we put forward in this book. And while we do so, we hope we'll heed our own cautions, and bear in mind the problems of these different types of study. We are, though, going to start with some international comparisons and, indeed, this is the very basis of our book. What is it about the French that protects them from heart disease?

2

THE FRENCH PARADOX

*'First need in the reform of hospital management?
That's easy! The death of all dietitians, and the resurrection of the French chef.'*
MARTIN H. FISCHER (1879-1962)

In the last chapter, we pointed out the enormous differences in rates of coronary heart disease around the world. But you don't have to look much further than the little corner of the world that is Western Europe to find some of the extremes in the figures. If we look at heart disease rates for 1989, Scotland and Northern Ireland fill the two top hotspots around the world, both in men and women, while France, Spain and Italy occupy three of the five places at the bottom of the table for all industrialized countries, including Japan.

A man in France has a risk of dying of coronary heart disease which is about one-third of that for a man in England, and one-quarter of that for a man in Scotland. A French woman's risk is one-fifth of that for a woman in England and one-eighth that of a Scottish woman.

But even if we look more closely at France, there are big differences. Head south across Europe and the risk goes down. Head south across France and the same applies. Coronary heart disease rates in Toulouse, in the south of France, are 30 per cent lower in men, and 50 per cent lower in women, than in Strasbourg or Lille, in the north. People in Lille or Strasbourg have more in common with their northern European neighbours than with

AGE-ADJUSTED DEATH RATE FROM HEART DISEASE PER 100,000 MEN AND WOMEN AGED 35-74 (1989)

COUNTRY	MEN	WOMEN
SCOTLAND	605	254
NORTHERN IRELAND	595	226
FORMER CZECHOSLOVAKIA	564	212
FINLAND	551	159
REPUBLIC OF IRELAND	514	201
HUNGARY	490	190
ENGLAND AND WALES	461	173
NEW ZEALAND	439	162
DENMARK	381	126
SWEDEN	350	104
USA	322	132
GERMANY	299	96
NETHERLANDS	297	89
LUXEMBOURG	280	76
SWITZERLAND	230	70
GREECE	224	73
ITALY	193	59
PORTUGAL	162	60
SPAIN	153	45
FRANCE	127	34
JAPAN	57	24

their Mediterranean compatriots, at least if you look inside their coronary arteries.

If we look at France as a whole, the coronary heart disease rates have a lot in common with many other Mediterranean countries. In Spain, Italy and Greece, death rates from coronary heart disease are universally low. As we mentioned in the last chapter, one of the earliest studies looking at national comparisons of heart disease rates was conducted by Ancel Keys, an American epidemiologist, in the 1960s. He found large differences in the seven countries studied. People living in Crete had rates about one-fifth of those in the United States. So what we are talking about is a general Mediterranean phenomenon and not particularly a French one. We'll come back to why the French are such a puzzle, and not the Cretans, in a moment.

Does this mean, then, that the French live for ever? Well, unfortunately, not quite! French men don't live much longer than English men because they have higher rates of accidents, liver disease and digestive diseases, as well as of some cancers. But French women do live longer than those in Britain, by three or four years. This is because they have lower rates of cancer, the other main cause of death, as well as heart disease. Which raises another question – if French men don't live any longer than men in the UK, could the differences in heart disease rates be artificial? Could they be the result of differences in the ways that doctors diagnose and label disease?

This is a question that has been addressed by MONICA, not a person but a project. It stands for a project to MONItor trends in CArdiovascular diseases, and was set up by the World Health Organization in the early 1980s. They have compared heart disease rates in twenty-one countries using standard sets of definitions. And MONICA has shown that problems of classification do not explain the low heart disease rates in France. According to MONICA, the French rates of coronary heart disease fit well with other Mediterranean countries, and not with their northern European neighbours.

In 1995, the world's oldest person, Jeanne Calment, celebrated her 120th birthday in Arles, in the south of France, where she has lived since she was a child. In a BBC report, she put her longevity down to using olive oil, drinking a little red wine ... and giving up smoking, which she did when she was 117.

What, then, is the paradox? And what do we mean by a paradox? A paradox is something that appears to be a contradiction but which is, in fact, true. It is defined in the Oxford Dictionary as 'a phenomenon that exhibits some conflict with preconceived notions of what is reasonable or possible'.

The picture opposite gives an example of a classic visual paradox – each section of the figure seems to make sense until you look at it as a whole. So what's the paradox about heart disease rates among French men and women?

The French Paradox is that, as a nation, the French have a high intake of animal fat and dairy products, very similar to those in the UK. They also share with the UK an average cholesterol level which is substantially higher than ideal, at around 6 mmol per litre. What's more, the cholesterol level in men and women living in Toulouse in southern France (see graphs on page 22) is somewhat higher than those in Strasbourg, in the north, despite the higher rates of heart disease in northern France. And because the French smoke as much as people in Britain, and have similar levels of blood pressure, these other two big risk factors aren't the answer either.

Here, then, is our paradox. It's a paradox because of our Diet-heart Model of coronary heart disease that we outlined in Chapter 1, and we show again here.

Animal fat ➤ Blood cholesterol ➤ Heart attacks

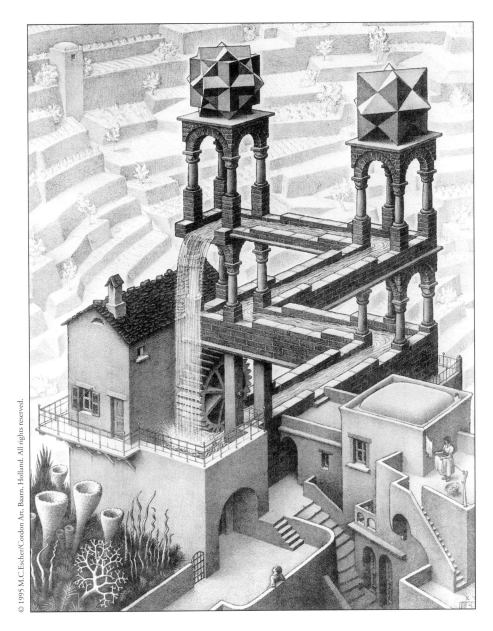

'The Waterfall' by MC Escher is a classic example of a visual paradox.

Despite a high intake of saturated fat (animal fats and dairy products), and cholesterol levels as high as in the UK, the French have only around one-third of the risk of heart attacks.

A paradox is a paradox only as long as the observation clashes with the preconceived notion. That's what makes the thing seem unreasonable or impossible. But to a scientist this is a challenge. There's no

COMPARISON OF DIFFERENT FACTORS AFFECTING RATE OF HEART DISEASE IN MEN AND WOMEN

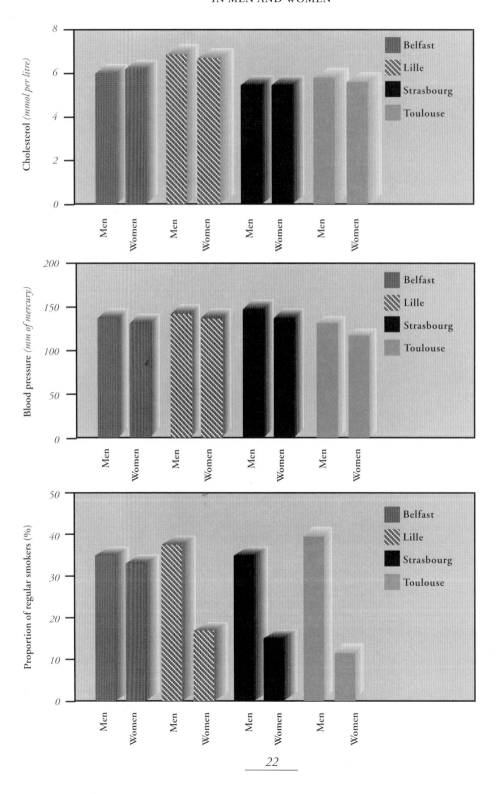

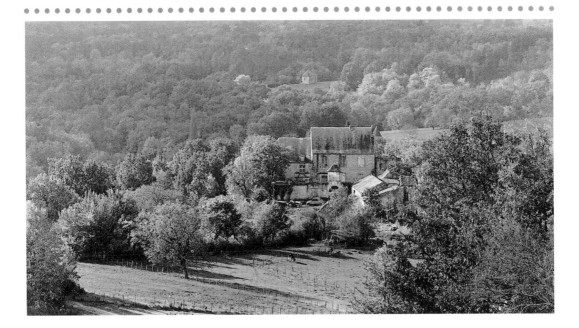

The people of the beautiful region of Dordogne

have low heart disease rates despite a diet rich

in animal fats.

such thing as absolute truth in science. If the preconceived notion doesn't fit the observation, and the observation is right, then the preconceived notion must be wrong.

What we are going to do for the rest of this book is to look at some of the explanations that have been proposed to explain the French Paradox. We've already adapted our Diet-heart Model, in the previous chapter, to make it look a little more flexible. And it's only that model, with animal fat and cholesterol in the centre, that makes the French Paradox a paradox. So when we find a new idea, and we feel that the observations hold water, we'll try to put together a new Diet-heart Model which will explain away the paradox of the French, perhaps by making animal fat and cholesterol less central to the new model.

We've already pointed out that the low rates of

coronary heart disease are not just a French phenomenon. Around the Mediterranean, coronary heart disease rates are uniformly low. In many of these countries, though, this is less of a surprise than in France. Animal fat intake is lower and so are people's cholesterol levels. But in the search for the solution to the French Paradox we may need to see if there are any clues around in the rest of the Mediterranean.

Let's start by having a quick glance at the similarities and the differences between what the British and the French eat and drink (see graph on page 24). The total fat intake is roughly similar in Britain and France, as is the intake of saturated, dairy and animal fats. But one of the big differences in the diet between the French and the British is in how the two populations get through fresh fruit and vegetables. In Britain we eat only about half as

DIFFERENCES BETWEEN THE FRENCH AND BRITISH DIET

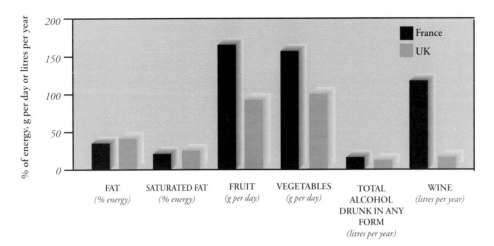

much fruit, and less than two-thirds of the fresh vegetables, that the French eat. Another difference is the amount of alcohol consumed. The French, on average, drink about 40 per cent more than people in the UK. But a much bigger contrast is in *what* they drink. Most alcohol in France is drunk as wine, but over 80 per cent of the alcohol drunk in Britain is as beer or spirits.

And herein may lie some of the answers to the French Paradox. We're going to concentrate on things we eat and drink, and the next five chapters will outline the candidates. They are, in the order we think most important:

olive oil;

fresh fruit and vegetables;

wine;

fish;

garlic, fibre and salt.

This book is about getting pleasure from eating good food and from drinking. Each chapter is not a homily about healthy lifestyles, but a set of ingredients to combine in recipes or meals as demonstrated by our cooks and wine expert in the remainder of the book.

3

OLIVE OIL: CANDIDATE I

'O Love, what hours were thine and mine,
In lands of palm and southern pine;
In lands of palm, of orange blossom,
Of olive, aloe, and maize and vine.'

THE DAISY; ALFRED, LORD TENNYSON

The paradox of the French is that, as a nation, they have a much lower risk of coronary heart disease than they should do. But the other paradox, which is perhaps even more interesting, is that not all French are equal. As we head south towards the Mediterranean, along the *Autoroute du Soleil* – the Motorway of the Sun – we are not only heading down through Europe, we're also heading down the table of heart disease rates in France. Can these north-south differences provide a clue? And is it important that it's not just the southern French, but the Italians, the Cretans and other Mediterranean people, who all have a lower chance of getting heart disease than people living in northern Europe?

In this chapter we're going to put the case for one of the major differences between people in the north of France and those in the south. And this difference is that the closer one gets to the Mediterranean, the more is olive oil used instead of butter. What's more, olive oil is also employed very widely all around the Mediterranean. Indeed, Ancel

Keys, one of the foremost scientists to study the question of diet and heart disease, pointed out that in Crete, it seems to be common to find 100-year-old farmers whose breakfast is often only a wine glass of olive oil.

So in this chapter, we'll explain why we think olive oil is healthy. A lot of the argument revolves around the cholesterol story – what it does explain and what it can't. In Chapter 1, we outlined the traditional Diet-heart Model, which is all based on cholesterol. And we tore into it fairly vigorously! But having knocked it down, are we going to try to put another cholesterol-based story back in its place? Well, we obviously can't abandon cholesterol completely. But we now have a much better idea than we had before about how cholesterol affects the arteries and the heart. In order to explain this, we're going to have to expand on some basic principles of biology and chemistry. So let's apologize in advance for taking you back to the classroom.

CHOLESTEROL – THE 'GOOD' AND THE 'BAD'

We've already introduced you to atherosclerosis, the thickening of the artery wall that leads to heart attacks. This damage is the result of the laying down of deposits of cholesterol in the artery walls. The cholesterol finds its way into these artery walls and then gets inside cells from the blood stream to make foam cells. But then these cells disappear, leaving behind large amounts of cholesterol sitting free in the artery wall as atherosclerotic plaques.

It's been known for a long time that the higher the level of cholesterol in the blood, the more is deposited in the arteries, and the higher the risk of heart attacks. This is clear not only from looking at rates of heart attacks and levels of cholesterol in different countries: those with the highest cholesterol levels generally have the highest risk of heart attacks. It's also seen in the information on heart attacks and cholesterol levels *within* any one population: people with the high levels get more heart attacks. But, as we've seen in Chapter 1, this relationship is not terribly strong. We pointed out that people with levels of cholesterol of around 7 mmol per litre have around a 50 per cent higher risk of heart attacks than people with levels of 6 mmol per litre.

Yet there's more information we can obtain from cholesterol levels about a person's risk. And this is because we now realize that cholesterol comes in two forms. These are known as high-density lipoprotein cholesterol (the 'good' cholesterol) and low-density lipoprotein cholesterol (the 'bad' cholesterol).

Cholesterol doesn't circulate around our bodies dissolved in our blood stream. Because it's a form of fat, if you tried to dissolve it in water, or in blood (which is 80 per cent water), it would be left floating. So cholesterol, like all the other fats in the blood stream, is carried around in the blood in little fatty particles. And these are held in emulsion, just like in emulsion paint. Or, perhaps more accurately,

like the fat in semi-skimmed milk, which makes up 2 per cent of its volume. If you shake up full cream milk and then leave it to stand, the cream separates out and floats to the top. But the fat in semi-skimmed milk, or in any of these emulsions, does not separate out on standing. This is because these tiny particles are very dispersed, and the emulsifiers which form their coats keep them suspended throughout the liquid.

Most of the cholesterol in our blood is carried in little globules called low-density lipoprotein (see opposite). Around half of the weight of each of these globules is made up of cholesterol. This is carried on the inside of the particle, away from the blood stream. And the globules are surrounded by a layer of protein and other chemicals, such as lecithin, which act as emulsifiers. The food industry has borrowed from the experiments of nature, and uses lecithin for just the same purpose – you'll notice it on the list of ingredients, for example, of drinking chocolate powder. This helps you stir it straight into cold milk, without the problems of trying to get your cocoa powder to dissolve!

Around a quarter of all the cholesterol in the blood is inside a completely different form of particle, called high-density lipoprotein (see opposite). These particles are much smaller than the low-density lipoprotein globules. They contain much less cholesterol and relatively more of the lining protein and emulsifiers. Because they contain less fat, they're more likely to sink than to float in watery solutions. And that's why they're called 'high-density'. The fact that they don't sink, though, is because of the emulsifiers.

Cholesterol doesn't just go round and round in the blood stream. It's in the circulation for a purpose. The cells in the body need access to different sorts of fats for two separate reasons. Fats are used as energy by the different tissues of the body (like the muscles, or the brain) but they also help in the process of making and repairing the cell walls or membranes. The lipoprotein particles carry fats around the body, so that fats which are made in one

STRUCTURE OF A LOW-DENSITY LIPOPROTEIN PARTICLE

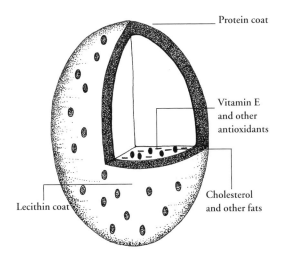

Protein coat

Vitamin E and other antioxidants

Cholesterol and other fats

Lecithin coat

STRUCTURE OF A HIGH-DENSITY LIPOPROTEIN PARTICLE

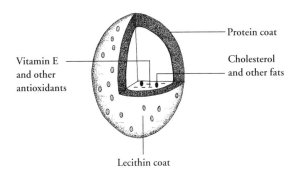

Protein coat

Cholesterol and other fats

Vitamin E and other antioxidants

Lecithin coat

reactions which transfer all the useful fat into the cells. As a waste product, it's left in the circulation, with cholesterol in it, until it is taken up by the liver. And it's there that its constituent parts are re-used. But while it's sitting in the blood stream, loaded with cholesterol and waiting to be removed, it can start doing damage. It is from these low-density lipoprotein particles that cholesterol gets into the walls of the blood vessels, which is the first step in atherosclerosis.

High-density lipoprotein is a very different particle altogether. The main job of this particle seems to be to suck cholesterol out of the wall of blood vessels, where it should never have been in the first place. And it's in the high-density lipoprotein particle that cholesterol is returned to the liver for re-use. So the two different particles have two very different, or even opposite, effects:

• the low-density lipoprotein carries cholesterol, which leaches into the walls of the artery to produce the atherosclerotic plaques;
• and the high-density lipoprotein sucks the cholesterol out of the artery wall.

In this way, low-density lipoprotein can be seen to be the 'bad' particle, and high-density lipoprotein the 'good' particle. And the cholesterol in low-density lipoprotein is bad because it is destined to cause atherosclerosis, while the cholesterol in high-density lipoprotein is coming out of the tissues around the body, where it was doing harm, and is heading back to the liver to be sorted out.

What has become clear is that if you have your cholesterol level measured, you get an answer made up of two types of cholesterol, both the cholesterol in low-density lipoprotein and cholesterol in high-density lipoprotein. Over the last twenty or so years, lots of studies have measured the two different sorts of cholesterol separately. When this is done, it's very clear that the higher one's level of low-density lipoprotein cholesterol, the higher one's risk of heart attacks, but the more

part of the body can reach other cells and tissues where they can be properly used. The fats that are absorbed through our intestines from the food we eat also need to get to other cells to be stored, or used as fuel.

Low-density lipoprotein is mostly a waste product – what's left at the end of a series of chemical high-density lipoprotein cholesterol one has, the lower that risk becomes. In other words, if the ratio of low-density lipoprotein to high-density lipoprotein is increased, either because of more of the first or less of the second, the risk of heart attacks is high. Conversely, if that ratio is low, either because of less of the 'bad' cholesterol or more of the 'good' one, then the risk of coronary heart disease is correspondingly reduced.

So are we now ready to look at the question of olive oil and butter? Well, at this stage, we can simply say that different sorts of fat and oil in the diet seem to have very different effects on both high-density and low-density lipoprotein cholesterol. But in order to explain this more clearly, we're afraid that we must go through another lesson.

FATTY ACIDS – SATURATED AND UNSATURATED

In Chapter 1 we have already mentioned the saturated and polyunsaturated fats and oils. But we've still not explained what they mean – just that animal fats are saturated and margarines polyunsaturated. In this section we're going to elaborate on this, so that the cholesterol story becomes clearer.

Animal fats – in milk, butter or fatty meat – are very similar chemicals to vegetable oils (sunflower oil, corn oil or peanut oil). Fats differ from oils by being solid, not liquid, at room temperature. But if you were to analyse the chemistry of lard or beef dripping, and of sunflower or olive oil, there would be more similarities than differences. Fats and oils all have a short backbone which is glycerol (or glycerine), a chemical that can be used, when purified, to make icing. Stuck on to this backbone are three long chains of carbon, hydrogen and oxygen, called fatty acids. The correct chemical name for the three fatty acids stuck together on a glycerol backbone is a triglyceride – literally three fatty acids and a glycerol. While the glycerol backbone is the same in any fat or oil, it's the fatty acids which are different and it's these differences which not only affect the temperature at

A TRIGLYCERIDE

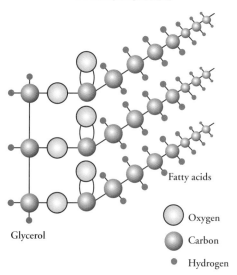

Fatty acids

○ Oxygen
● Carbon
• Hydrogen

Glycerol

which the fat or the oil melts; the different fatty acids also play a major role in affecting levels of cholesterol, and also other aspects of the chemistry of cholesterol, which we will come to later.

Animal fats, whether in dairy products such as butter or cheese, or in the fat in meat, contain almost entirely saturated fatty acids. These fatty acids are long, straight chains, with the carbon atoms joined together by single links, or bonds.

A SATURATED FATTY ACID

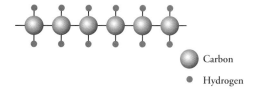

● Carbon
• Hydrogen

In vegetable oils, such as sunflower or olive oil, the fatty acids look a little different. In one or more places along the chain of carbon atoms, there are the unsaturated, double links, or bonds, between two adjacent carbons.

While at first sight putting a double link between two atoms would seem to make it stronger, in fact it has rather the opposite effect. Imagine the

AN UNSATURATED FATTY ACID

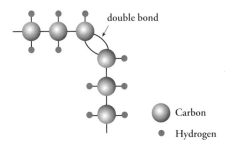

double bond

Carbon

Hydrogen

A MONOUNSATURATED FATTY ACID

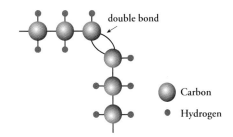

double bond

Carbon

Hydrogen

A POLYUNSATURATED FATTY ACID

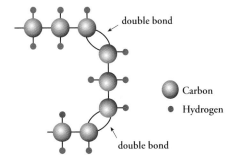

double bond

Carbon

Hydrogen

double bond

carbon links in the fatty acid as we show them in the diagram of the unsaturated fatty acid above. You'll see that the two links of a double bond have the effect of producing distortion, one on the other. The consequence is that several different chemical reactions are able to produce a break in one of the two links. We'll return to this property of the unsaturated bonds in two places later in this book. The first will be to talk about the manufacture of margarine and shortening by hydrogenation, which comes later in this chapter. But we'll also be discussing the whole question of oxidation, free radicals and antioxidants which we look at in detail in Chapter 4.

Besides the question of stability, there's another effect of putting one or more of these double bonds in a fatty acid. When three unsaturated fatty acids link up with a glycerol backbone, the melting point of that oil is lower and it becomes liquid at room temperature. Which is why, as we've said, saturated fatty acids make fats, and unsaturated ones make oils.

Just a few more points to make before this chemistry lesson ends! The first point is that in vegetable oils, there can be anything between one and four unsaturated, double bonds in each of the fatty acids which make up the triglycerides. If the fatty acid contains just one double bond it's called monounsaturated. But if it contains more than one, it's called polyunsaturated.

These are terms which you've no doubt heard many times over. And if you haven't done so yet,

you soon will have, because we'll be coming back to them a fair amount, both in this chapter and later in the book.

The second point is that we use a sort of shorthand: a saturated fat is one containing saturated fatty acids, and a polyunsaturated one contains polyunsaturated fatty acids.

The final point is that in most polyunsaturated vegetable oils, the first unsaturated, double link, or bond, is six carbon atoms up from the end of the carbon chain furthest away from the glycerol. There's the mystery clue – don't forget it! Just as in an Agatha Christie mystery, it might appear totally without logic or relevance at the moment, but we'll remind you of it again in Chapter 6 when we start talking about fish.

The group of fatty acids which are going to have a very high profile in this book are called monounsaturated. These have just one solitary double

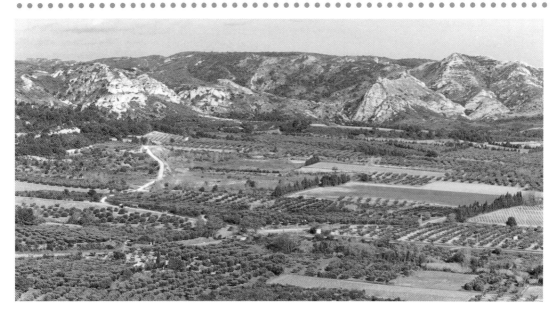

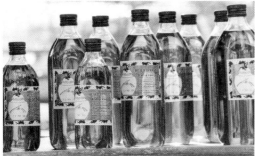

As we go further south in France,

the abundance of olive groves is reflected

in their choice of oil for cooking.

bond in the chain of carbon atoms. But what is most surprising is that fatty acids in this class have effects which are very different either from saturated fatty acids – which differ by having just one less double bond – or from polyunsaturated fatty acids – with just one more double bond.

THE FAT WE EAT AND OUR RISK OF HEART DISEASE

We come back to the major study made by Ancel Keys about thirty years ago, looking at heart disease risk in seven different countries around the world. The results showed huge differences in the rates of heart disease between different countries, with people in Japan or Crete being substantially less vulnerable than those, say, in the United States. The investigators of this study came up with a series of differences in the diets in these countries which they related to the range of heart disease rates. To start with, they found no link whatsoever between the total amount of fat included in the diet in different nations and the rates of coronary heart disease. In fact, in these seven countries, the highest fat intake was found in Crete, which had one of the lowest rates of heart disease. But other countries like Japan, with a very low risk of heart disease, had a diet which was extremely low in fat. You will note, by the way, that when used in this sense, the term 'fats' is an abbreviation for all fats and oils in the diet.

Are all animal fats equal?

We tend to think fairly glibly of all animal fats being equal, but this may well not be true. Some may be more equal than others. Animal fats from most sources contain saturated fatty acids. But the saturated fatty acids in butter and other dairy products have more of an influence on cholesterol levels – in particular the 'bad', low-density lipoprotein cholesterol – than the fatty acids in fatty meat. If this is so, then dairy produce may be worse for the heart than red meat – though this must remain highly speculative for the time being. And yet if this is true, perhaps the French are even more of a paradox, because they have a huge amount of their animal fat as cheese, crème fraîche and butter. But it's also possible that the process of converting milk and cream into cheese does something to the fatty acids which makes them less harmful. The jury is still out on this.

RELATIONSHIP BETWEEN SATURATED FAT
AND CORONARY HEART DISEASE IN MEN IN
THE SEVEN COUNTRIES STUDY
UNDERTAKEN IN THE 1960S

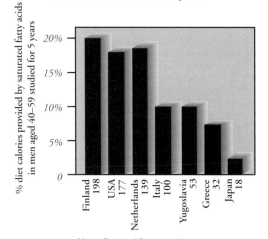

Heart disease risk per 10,000 men per year

But the Seven Countries Study came up with enormous differences in the dietary levels of saturated fat. And there was a direct link between saturated fat intake and coronary heart disease in the centres studied in these seven countries. So in general, high-risk populations ate as much as four times more animal and dairy fats than were eaten in low-risk areas, and had around four times higher death rates from coronary heart disease. The diagram from the Seven Countries Study is shown above. It links the intake of animal and dairy fat with coronary heart disease rates.

Several other more recent studies have done similar analyses, either for animal fats as a whole or just for dairy fat, and have all come up with similar answers. The graph on page 20 shows results from seventeen countries, including France, using

information collected on dairy fat intake twenty years after the Seven Countries Study.

Again there's a strong link between national dairy fat intake and national heart disease rates. But this graph also shows France as an exception – this nation has a lower rate of heart disease than would be expected from a number of different standpoints, including dairy fat intake.

The other thing the Seven Countries Study came up with was the link between dietary intake of fats and oils in different populations, their serum cholesterol levels, and their heart disease rates. Indeed, we could even suggest that the Seven Countries Study was one of the main reasons why the traditional Diet-heart Model which we pulled to pieces in Chapter 1 gained such a following. The formulae put together by Ancel Keys linked coronary heart disease rates to intakes of saturated and unsaturated fats, and also related dietary fat intake to levels of cholesterol. In this way, the study came up with the conclusion that a high intake of animal fat and dairy produce results in a higher level of serum cholesterol, which in turn produces a higher risk of heart disease. Conversely, a

RELATIONSHIP BETWEEN DEATH RATES FROM HEART DISEASE AND DAIRY FAT INTAKE
(—— = estimate of expected rate of heart disease at any level of dairy fat intake)

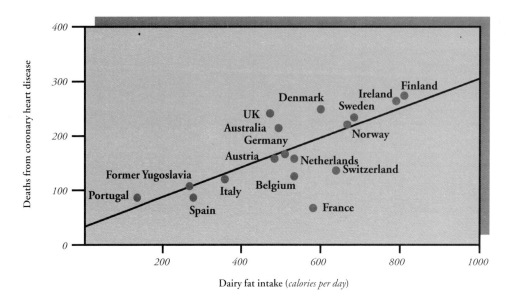

Dairy fat intake (*calories per day*)

high intake of polyunsaturated fat (or oil) is linked with lower levels of serum cholesterol and lower rates of heart disease.

What, then, is the problem with the Seven Countries Study? If it really *is* possible to come up with an equation that can tell us how our diet affects our level of cholesterol, and how both of these affect our risk of heart disease, why shouldn't we change our diets accordingly? There are two main problems.

Firstly the Seven Countries Study did not measure high-density lipoprotein and low-density lipoprotein cholesterol separately. This means that a 'low cholesterol' could be low either because of lower levels of the 'bad' cholesterol or of the 'good' one. Secondly, the huge differences in cholesterol levels and in heart disease rates seen in populations from different countries, and which relate to the dietary patterns in those countries, are just not seen to anything like the same extent *within* the population of a single country. The formulae seem to fit better with populations than with people.

> ### What about cholesterol intake?
>
> *Cholesterol is found in most of the foods which contain saturated fat, and also in fairly high amounts in eggs. Keys' equations included dietary cholesterol intake, as well as that of saturated fat, among the predictors of coronary heart disease rates. But variations in the intake of cholesterol go hand in hand with differences in the amount of animal fat in the diet. This means that it is extremely difficult to separate out any individual contribution from cholesterol intake – on heart disease rates or on cholesterol levels. Other approaches suggest that, certainly as far as cholesterol levels in the blood are concerned, the effects of changing the amount of cholesterol in the diet are relatively small.*

Let's look, then, at the relationship of saturated and unsaturated fat intake with levels of 'good' and 'bad' cholesterol in the circulation. And also at some of the studies of diet and heart disease rates in individual populations.

A number of studies have tried to look at the relationship of heart disease to people's diet within a population. These studies have found a convincing, but fairly weak, link between intake of animal fats, and that of cholesterol, and heart disease rates in these individuals.

As a separate approach, people have looked at the effect of cutting down the amount of saturated fat in the diet and comparing the development of heart disease with that in a group of people whose diets have not changed. Many studies have now appeared, and overall they have shown that the people put on a low-fat diet developed about 7 per cent less heart disease. But the only one where there was any major benefit tackled other risk factors, such as smoking, as well.

RISK OF CORONARY HEART DISEASE OVER 19 YEARS IN 1900 MEN ACCORDING TO THEIR INTAKE OF SATURATED FAT

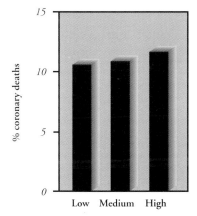

Intake of saturated fat as a proportion of total calories

How can it be, then, that saturated fats might be bad for you, but cutting down the amount of animal fat in the diet doesn't lessen your risk of con-

tracting heart disease? Part of the problem, at least, might be the realization that cholesterol is not just simply cholesterol, but either 'good' or 'bad' cholesterol. If we think of how we would react if someone told us to cut down the amount of saturated fat in our diet, our instinct would be to think what we could put in its place. If we can't use butter, then we'll use margarine. If we can't cook in lard, we'll use cooking oil. So most thinking about saturated fat reduction over the years has been about substituting polyunsaturated for saturated fat. If someone who has a lot of animal fat and dairy produce in their diet substitutes polyunsaturated oils (such as corn oil) for fats in the cooking, and uses soft margarine (instead of butter), their total fat intake will be exactly the same as before. What will be different is that they'll be having a higher ratio of polyunsaturated to saturated fatty acids. Several studies have looked at how such a change affects cholesterol level in the blood. And they show that such a substitution reduces the levels of 'bad', low-density lipoprotein cholesterol by around 10 per cent of the total. But they also have an effect on the 'good', high-density lipoprotein cholesterol, and by around the same amount. And if the 'bad' cholesterol levels fall by around 10 per cent, and the 'good' cholesterol levels fall by around 10 per cent, what's the net effect on the ratio of 'bad' to 'good' cholesterol? Of course, absolutely none!

We've already spent some time knocking the cholesterol story, but it's still worth making a point. Even if the cholesterol story were true, and that low-density lipoprotein cholesterol and its ratio to high-density lipoprotein cholesterol explained everything there is about coronary heart disease, simply substituting vegetable oils for animal fats in our diet would be unlikely to have any effect.

But it's also worth throwing in another thought, to put another spoke in this wheel. Just because exchanging vegetable oil for animal fat doesn't improve the cholesterol, this is not the same as saying animal fat is okay. As we pointed out in Chapter 1, there's some suggestion that a high intake of animal fat can have an effect on the risk of heart attacks not through any influence on atherosclerosis but by making the blood more sticky, and so more likely to clot. But on the other hand, as we will see in Chapter 4, polyunsaturated fats may be harmful for the blood vessels because they may affect the way cholesterol is handled, making 'bad' cholesterol even worse, by a process called oxidation. But that is another story.

One final thought about the possible merits or risks of simply substituting margarine for butter. There's a suspicion from one or two reports that a high intake of polyunsaturated fat may increase the risk of gall bladder disease. But, to set against this, there's an enormous amount of evidence that a diet containing a lot of animal fat and meat is associated with an increased risk of cancer of the colon and perhaps also of the breast.

> ### So what have we said?
>
> *Replacing animal fat with polyunsaturates: lowers 'good' as well as 'bad' cholesterol; may lower blood stickiness; hasn't been shown to have a major effect on heart attacks in most studies; may reduce the risk of some cancers but increase that of gall bladder disease.*

And so what can we conclude from this? Should we be eating butter or should we be eating margarine? Let's look again at the Nurses' Health Study.

DOES MARGARINE PROTECT FROM HEART DISEASE?

We've already introduced the Nurses' Health Study in Chapter 2. Around 20 years ago some 121,700 female nurses in the United States completed detailed questionnaires about their diet, their health and their lifestyle. This provided the opportunity to look at the risk of developing a whole col-lection of different diseases in the ensuing years according to what that person usually eats, at least as recorded on that single dietary questionnaire.

When the rates of heart disease were compared in women eating different amounts of margarine, a surprising result emerged. Women having more than four portions of margarine, each of about one teaspoon per day, had around 66 per cent greater risk of developing heart disease than women who had margarine less than once a month. In other words, there was a clear relationship between high margarine intake and the risk of heart disease. In the same nurses, there was absolutely no relationship between the amount of meat in the diet, or that of butter, and the risk of heart attacks.

So what is it about margarine, or maybe particularly American margarine, that might be harmful? Professor Walter Willett, the leading investigator in the Nurses' Health Study, thinks that it's a new and evil monster lurking out there: trans fatty acids. So just when you thought you'd met all the players in the game, along comes another one, and one holding a smoking gun. But before we can decide whether the evidence is enough to convict, we need to find out a bit more about the profile of this suspected culprit, where it comes from, and why it might be harmful.

Trans fatty acids are found in small amounts in nature, but they are produced in much larger amounts in the processing of food. The reason for their emergence comes from the fact that polyunsaturated fatty acids, which make up the vegetable oils, melt at a very low temperature, so they're liquid not only at room temperature but also in the fridge. This makes it necessary for the manufacturers to do something to make them more easily handled and packaged. Hence the process of hydrogenation, or hardening. And in addition, hydrogenated oils have a longer shelf life because they are less likely to go rancid.

The technique of hydrogenation was discovered at the beginning of the twentieth century. If a vegetable oil is warmed in the presence of hydrogen, most or all of the double bonds are converted to the much more stable single-bond form. This occurs by the hydrogen being sucked into the fatty acid and breaking one half of the double bond. If a polyunsaturated fatty acid is completely hydrogenated, every unsaturated bond becomes saturated. And that will make the polyunsaturated fatty acid into a saturated one. But if all the double bonds except one become saturated, then the fatty acid with the solitary double bond is called a monounsaturated fatty acid.

TRANS FATTY ACIDS FORMING DURING THE PROCESS OF HYDROGENATION

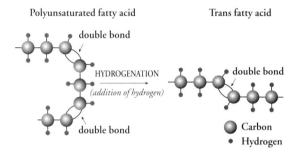

Monounsaturated fatty acids occur in nature, as we'll be discussing at some length later in this chapter. But the naturally occurring monounsaturated fatty acid looks very different from the one produced by hydrogenating vegetable oils. This is because of the way in which the long chain of carbons lines up. In nature the double bond creates a sort of fold in the carbon chain, so that the fatty acid doubles back on itself. The chemists call this a cis fatty acid (see above right), implying that the two chains are on the same side of the molecule.

When a polyunsaturated fatty acid is hydrogenated in all except one of the double bonds, the carbon chain folds on itself in the opposite way. And now the fatty acid lies in a completely straight line, except for the zig-zag in the middle of it created by the remaining unsaturated bond. Because the two carbon chains are going away from each other on either side of the double bond, this is called a trans fatty acid, meaning opposite (see above right).

CIS AND TRANS FATTY ACIDS

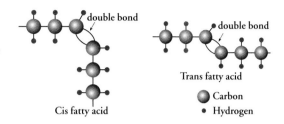

Hydrogenation of vegetable oils made a dramatic impact on the amount of trans fatty acids in the diet. In the early part of the century, hydrogenation was used mainly to turn oils into vegetable shortening because this was a great deal cheaper than animal fats or lard. But this shortening contained about one-third or more of its fatty acids as trans fatty acids rather than either polyunsaturated or saturated ones. More recently, the emphasis has been on cutting down animal fat intake, and substituting it with margarine. Between the 1960s and early 1980s, much of the margarine being eaten, both in Britain and the United States, was hard margarine. And this, too, contained a high proportion of trans fatty acids. But also several of the fast food chains, particularly in the United States, stopped using beef fat for frying. Instead they cooked in hydrogenated oils, which contain up to one-third of trans fatty acids.

Surprisingly, trans fatty acids have very different effects on cholesterol levels from those of any of its close relatives. Several studies have looked at what happens when people swap either trans fatty acids or saturated fat for the natural, cis forms, of the monounsaturated fats (see graph overleaf). These studies agree that the trans fatty acids raise the levels of 'bad', low-density lipoprotein cholesterol similarly to saturated fats. But disturbingly, they also lower the levels of the 'good', high-density lipoprotein cholesterol. So as a result, the ratio of 'bad' to 'good' cholesterol goes up even more than it does by eating a similar amount of saturated fat.

So why should trans fatty acids be so harmful? It

EFFECT OF DIFFERENT DIETS ON THE RATIO OF LOW-DENSITY TO HIGH-DENSITY LIPOPROTEIN

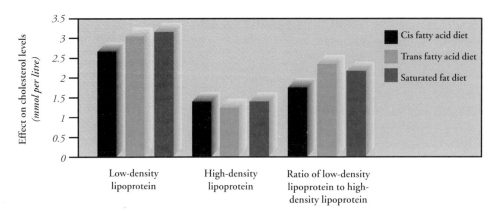

may have something to do with their chemical structure. If we lie together a model of the four different sorts of molecules, a saturated fatty acid, a trans monounsaturated fatty acid, a cis monounsaturated fatty acid and a polyunsaturated fatty acid, we can see that the two that look the most alike are the saturated and the trans monounsaturated acids.

COMPARISON OF THE DIFFERENT TYPES OF FATTY ACID

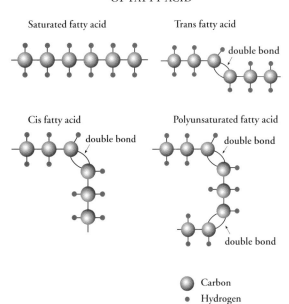

So is it the trans fatty acids in the margarines that explain the findings of the Nurses' Health Study? This may well be the case. Walter Willett looked not only at the nurses' intake of butter, animal fat and margarine, but at the total amount of trans fatty acid from hydrogenated vegetable oils and shortening. And there was a clear link of heart disease risk to the amount of trans fatty acids eaten. People who had more than 3 per cent of their total daily calories from trans fatty acids had around 80 per cent higher risk of heart attacks than those who had half of this intake or less.

How relevant is this to what happens in the United Kingdom? This must remain an unanswered question. Much more of the margarine in Britain is spread-straight-from-the-fridge type margarine, and not hard margarine. What's more, the Americans are much fonder of their muffins and doughnuts than the British, so have a lot more hydrogenated vegetable oils as shortening. They also eat out, in fast food chains and burger bars, more than people do in Britain. For all these reasons, we can work out that the average British diet contains only around a half as much trans fatty acids as is eaten in the United States. And a European study looking at trans fatty acids and heart attack risk in nine countries found very weak links – perhaps because in general the intake is below the danger levels in Europe.

But, however unjustified the concern, the food industry is beginning to respond to these anxieties. They are beginning to make soft margarines containing much fewer trans fatty acids. As a result, you will notice the 'low in trans' logo on the packets of many of the soft margarines.

So how much more complicated can it get? We have slammed the saturates and lambasted the polyunsaturates. And now we've found a new culprit. Not only that, but it's lurking in the very food that many of the 'experts' have been telling us for years that we should be eating: polyunsaturated margarines. And if we can't eat butter and we can't eat margarine, what's left?

The glib answer, of course, is that we ought to be cutting down on the amount of fat we eat anyway. Fat is full of calories, so cutting down on fat will help to prevent gaining weight. We've also given you some evidence that high fat intake, of one variety, may cause not only heart disease but cancer and, of the other variety, gall bladder disease. And with the polyunsaturates come the trans fatty acids, with all their bad press. But, as you may have forgotten, since we have not mentioned it for a while, this chapter is about olive oil. And olive oil, with what it contains, may be the key to many mysteries: the French Paradox; long life in Crete; and also the question of what we are left with if we say no to butter and no to margarine.

OLIVE OIL – RICH IN MONOUNSATURATES AND GOOD FOR HEALTH

The olive tree, with its characteristic silvery green leaves, grows widely all over southern France, Italy, Greece and Spain. Olive trees may live for a hundred or more years, and they develop intricate patterns of twisting and intertwining of their trunks and branches. The wood of these trees can be carved to make delicately grained bowls and ornaments.

Olives are widely used for their oil. Olive oil is viewed as the queen of all oils by many chefs in most Mediterranean countries, particularly for salads but also in cooking. In France, olive oil is widely used in the south, but much less commonly so in the north. In fact, as you travel south through France, starting from the rich pastures of Normandy, the big industrial city of Lille, or the Vosges mountains of Alsace – heavily influenced in style, language and cooking by the Germans – one moves away from the land of cooking in butter to the land of olive oil. And as we've already seen, the north-south gradient in heart disease runs parallel to the butter-olive oil divide.

Olive oil is not solely a French phenomenon. Quite the contrary! In Crete, where Ancel Keys noted one of the lowest rate of heart disease in the Seven Countries Study, he remarked that this may have been because of their high intake of olive oil. In that study the Cretans had one of the lowest intakes of animal fat in any group studied. But, remarkably, their total fat consumption was hardly any different from the northern European nations such as Finland – because they ate so much olive oil. In Italy, the olive is widely respected as a source of the most exquisite, and most expensive, olive oil available. Sit down to a meal in a restaurant in Italy, and you are more likely to be given a bowl of olive oil to dip your bread in than a dish of butter.

The best olive oil is extracted from hand-picked olives – which stops the fruit getting bruised if it's allowed to fall. Ripe olives are black, and when they are pressed they produce sweet light-golden olive oil, which the French use in large amounts. In Italy, olives are more commonly picked when they are still green, and not fully ripe. This makes olive oil which is slightly sharper and richer in flavour. The best oils come from what is called 'cold pressing'. This means that during the processing, in which stones are used to grind the olives and press the pulp, no heat or water is used. And the final factor which makes a huge difference to the quality of the product is whether that oil comes from the first pressing of the olive, or a later pressing. So the very

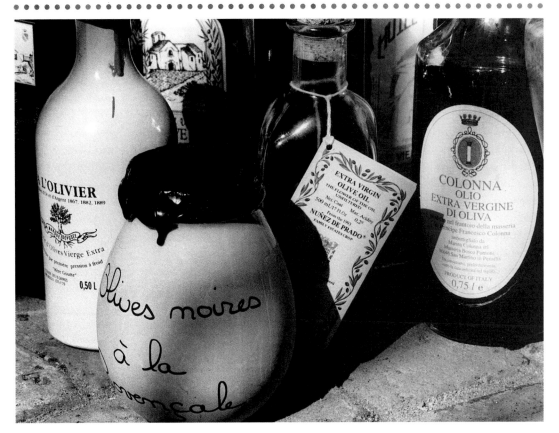

There can be almost as much variety in the flavour

and price of a bottle of olive oil as there is in

a bottle of red wine.

best oils – from the highest quality, hand-picked olives, from the first pressing, and preferably cold-pressed – are known as 'extra virgin' olive oil. Later pressings, or oil from less high quality olives, can still be called 'virgin' oil – there are obviously sub-categories of virginity! But if made from pulp left over from earlier pressings, along with skins and pips, it's known just as 'pure' olive oil.

Olive oil is rich in a type of fatty acid which we have met earlier in this chapter, but only briefly. The monounsaturated fatty acid makes up some 70 per cent of all fatty acids in olive oil. You may remember that the monounsaturated fatty acid has this name because it has just one unsaturated, or double, bond. This is in contrast to the two or more unsaturated bonds in polyunsaturated fatty acids and the complete lack of them in the saturated ones. But we also brought up the notion of hydro-genation or hardening, to convert the liquid polyunsaturated fatty acids into more solid fats dur-ing processing. In this conversion, it's often the case that polyunsaturated fatty acids are left only partly hydrogenated, with just one single unsaturated bond. But as we pointed out, this is often in the unnatural trans shape, as we show in the diagram on page 35. By contrast, the naturally occurring monounsaturated fatty acids usually lie in the cis shape. This means that both ends of the fatty acid, on the opposite sides of the double bond, face the same way. If they go in opposite directions, that's the trans fatty acid.

Olive oil is the richest source of monounsaturated fatty acids, but certainly not the only one. Other oils also contain a smaller, but still large proportion of monounsaturated fatty acids. And bearing in mind the cost of olive oil, we'll be returning to this question a little later.

Some of these oils are very cheap and could easily be considered for everyday cooking. Rapeseed oil, for example is low in cost, and is rapidly getting a good, and healthy, reputation. Some of the others are really very specialist. Walnut oil, for

example, has a rich, nutty flavour and, when cold pressed, is a delicious way to enhance the flavour of a green salad.

Monounsaturated fatty acids – what do they do?

We've already seen the problems with polyunsaturated fats – if we substitute them for saturated ones, they may lower the cholesterol level, but only by lowering both the 'good' and the 'bad'. We've also seen that a lot of the fats that are made by processing polyunsaturated fats to make them suitable for spreads and baking involve hydrogenation or hardening. And that this change produces the trans fatty acid – which ups the levels of 'bad', low-density lipoprotein cholesterol and drops that of the 'good', high-density lipoprotein cholesterol.

Fatty acid composition of some common oils and fats

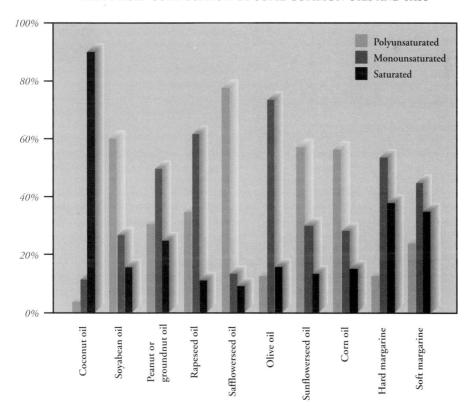

So, what do monounsaturated fatty acids do? Several researchers have looked at what happens when people change their diets from being high in either saturated or polyunsaturated fat, simply swapping to monounsaturated fat instead.

COMPARISON OF THE EFFECTS OF MONOUNSATURATED AND POLYUNSATURATED DIETS ON LOW-DENSITY AND HIGH-DENSITY LIPOPROTEIN CHOLESTEROL

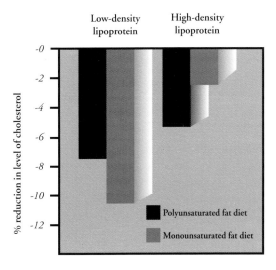

What is clear from all of these studies is that monounsaturated fats are extremely good at lowering levels of the 'bad', low-density lipoprotein cholesterol. In this regard, they are just as effective as the polyunsaturated fats. But the big difference is in what they do to the 'good', high-density lipoprotein cholesterol. While the diet high in polyunsaturated fats lowers these levels, the high monounsaturated fat diet has virtually no effect at all. As a result, the ratio of 'bad', low-density lipoprotein to 'good', high-density lipoprotein cholesterol gets better to an important degree with monounsaturated fats but not at all by diets rich in polyunsaturated fats (see graph above).

There may also be other good effects from a high monounsaturated fat diet. As we'll see in Chapter 4, other chemical changes, called oxidation, can happen to the cholesterol particles, which make them more likely to produce atherosclerosis. A diet high in monounsaturated fats may have a useful effect here too. There are also some clues suggesting that olive oil, or other monounsaturated fats, can improve levels of blood sugar in people with diabetes.

Finally, it's not just the damage to the wall of the blood vessel which can be reduced by monounsaturated fats like olive oil, as we'll see in this next section.

MONOUNSATURATED FATS – CAN THEY INFLUENCE THE RISK OF BLOOD CLOTTING IN THE CORONARY ARTERY?

A lot of what we've spent our time talking about so far connects the things we eat to the amount of cholesterol being deposited in the walls of our blood vessels. But as we've already said, a heart attack is not just hardening of the arteries. The attack itself requires something extra to happen to that damaged artery wall. The cholesterol plaque may burst, and this allows blood in, so that a big 'blister' grows and the vessel becomes blocked. Alternatively, blood might be able to clot on the roughened and irregular wall of a narrowed artery even without the plaque bursting. It's not fully clear which of these processes is usually the main player in producing a heart attack. But when someone has already had one heart attack, we believe that the blood-clotting mechanisms play a very important role in their risk of having another one. This is why half an aspirin tablet every day is so valuable in most people after a heart attack – it reduces the stickiness of the blood clotting cells, the platelets.

A group of doctors from Lyon, in south-east France, led by Professor Serge Renaud, have long been interested in the mechanisms that underlie the French Paradox. They reasoned that these mechanisms could work either through the risk of the artery wall thickening with cholesterol, or that of blood clotting. And they have recently done a very intriguing study. They took just over 600 men and women who had recently had a heart attack. Half of them were put on a Mediterranean-type diet, with an increase in the amount of fish, fruit and vegetables, more bread and less meat. But the main change was in the sort of oil and fat they ate. Because the people were not happy to use just olive oil, they were given instead a special margarine made mainly from rapeseed oil. This oil, like olive oil, is very rich in monounsaturated fatty acids. The other half of the patients were not given any special dietary advice – they were given health education the same as anyone who has had a heart attack.

Over the next two years, in spite of the difference in diet between the two groups of patients, there was absolutely no difference seen in the levels of cholesterol – either 'good' or 'bad'. But there was a dramatic effect on recurrent heart attacks. Of 302 people on the Mediterranean diet:

- three died of a heart attack;
- five had a second heart attack but survived.

While of 303 people on the usual diet:
- sixteen died of a heart attack;
- seventeen had a second heart attack but survived.

In other words, this diet was able to reduce the risk of recurrent heart attacks by over 70 per cent without producing any change in the cholesterol level.

This research is interesting for a whole number of reasons. Firstly, this study suggests that it's never too late to start eating a healthy diet. Secondly, it gives a clue that blood clotting mechanisms are very important in explaining the benefits of the Mediterranean diet. Even though the cholesterol levels didn't change, these people were over 70 per cent protected from heart attacks by the diet – and in a fairly short period of time. The third reason it's important is that it suggests a cheap and healthy alternative for olive oil in everyday cooking and eating.

Rapeseed oil comes from the yellow flowers grown in increasing profusion across the fields of England and the rest of Europe. In France, the plant is grown for animal feed, not for oil for human consumption. Nevertheless, rapeseed oil is high in monounsaturates – second only to olive oil in the league table. And, as we will see in Chapter 6, rapeseed oil also contains a fatty acid called alpha-linolenic acid, which may share with fish oil a particular advantage in terms of stopping blood clotting.

To summarize

What we have said in this chapter is pretty complicated. We've pointed out that the 'bad', low-density lipoprotein cholesterol is one of several factors which damage the artery wall to cause atherosclerosis. And another form of cholesterol, the 'good', high-density lipoprotein cholesterol, protects the vessel wall. We have discussed the fact that animal fat is one of the influences on the 'bad', low-density lipoprotein cholesterol levels. And it seems that a diet high in saturated fats can increase the risk of heart attack not just through cholesterol levels but through other mechanisms – perhaps to do with blood clotting. Substituting animal fat with polyunsaturated fat, as found in most vegetable oils, lowers the levels of both 'bad', low-density lipoprotein cholesterol and 'good', high-density lipoprotein cholesterol, which means that it produces no net effect on the ratio of 'bad' to 'good' cholesterol.

However, it isn't fully clear whether such a change in diet has any overall effect on the rate of heart attacks. Some studies show minor effects, although people eating lots of margarine don't appear to be protected from heart disease. What is obvious is that processing of oils into shortening and margarine produces trans fatty acids. And these have bad effects on both sorts of cholesterol – the 'good' goes down and the 'bad' goes up, with what, in large amounts, may be parallel effects on the risk of heart attacks.

A NEW MODEL LINKING DIET WITH HEART DISEASE

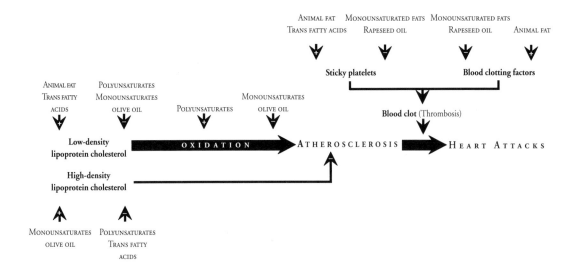

THE EFFECTS OF CHANGES IN INTAKE OF DIFFERENT TYPES OF FATTY ACIDS ON CHOLESTEROL LEVELS AND HEART ATTACK RISKS

	EFFECTS ON:			
Type of fatty acid	'Bad', low-density lipoprotein cholesterol	'Good', high-density lipoprotein cholesterol	Ratio of 'bad' to 'good' cholesterol	Heart attacks
SATURATED	↑	–	↑	↑
POLYUNSATURATED	↓	↓	→	?
TRANS	↑	↓	↑↑	↑
MONOUNSATURATED	↓	–	↓	↓

If, however, saturated fats in the diet are replaced by monounsaturated fats, levels of 'bad', low-density lipoprotein cholesterol go down, without any ill effect on the 'good', high-density lipoprotein cholesterol (or, of course, the ratio). In addition, blood stickiness seems to be strongly benefited by a monounsaturated fat diet.

What does this mean as far as reducing heart attack risk is concerned? As far as fat is concerned, it means, firstly, reducing the overall amount of fat, especially saturated fat, in the diet; and, secondly, substituting monounsaturated fat for part of the saturated fat which is being removed.

So how can we summarize this chapter? Not in scientific terms but in the way we think about food and cooking? We agree with most of the experts – the sort of diet many people are eating is not healthy. It contains much too much animal fat and dairy produce. We don't think fatty cuts of meat are healthy, especially if the fat is not allowed a chance to melt off, or is not cut off before or after cooking. But we can understand being extremely partial to a nice roast leg of lamb, or a grilled steak. Just use a little bit of olive oil for basting or grilling, having cut off most of the fat.

As to the butter or margarine argument, perhaps the most important message is 'less of whichever'. Several of the soft margarine manufacturers are taking the trans story very seriously. And a number of them are also using more and more monounsaturated fatty acids, such as olive oil, in margarines. It won't be long, though, before other sorts of margarines are available – like the one that was used in the Lyon study of patients after heart attacks, which was made with monounsaturate-rich rapeseed oil. And that will provide spreads with lower levels of saturated and trans fatty acids, and more monounsaturated fatty acids, than we've had before.

For cooking, try rapeseed oil or groundnut oil instead of corn oil. For salads, or for tossing vegetables, just experiment with the different sort of olive oils around. They are certainly expensive compared to corn oil, but you're not using them for deep-frying chips! Let's recommend something else which is worth a try – a drizzle of olive oil on a slice of toast or a bagel. There are so many wonderful flavours of oils, from Spain, France, Italy or Greece, that can be teamed with any one of several dozen different sorts of loaf. And if you try this, you'll be using much smaller amounts of olive oil than butter, so the price will actually be quite similar.

THE NUTRITIONAL CONTENT OF SOME MONOUNSATURATED SPREADS

Per 100 g	OLIVIO Reduced fat spread suitable for cooking/ frying	OLIVITE Low-fat spread not suitable for baking/frying	ST IVEL MONO Rapeseed oil spread suitable for baking/ shallow frying	OLIVE GOLD Reduced fat spread suitable for baking
CALORIES	544	360	675	545
FAT	60 g	39.9 g	75 g	60 g
SATURATES	11 g	9 g	11.5 g	13.8 g
MONOUNSATURATES	29 g	19.6 g	35 g	34.2 g
POLYUNSATURATES	13 g	5.2 g	14.7 g	12 g

4

FRUIT AND VEGETABLES: CANDIDATE 2

'An apple a day keeps the doctor away.'
PROVERB

People in France have a very different attitude to fruit and vegetables from, for example, the British. To start with, the average French person's diet has around 60 per cent more vegetables than that of someone in the United Kingdom. They also eat around twice as much fruit, and just like the butter and olive oil story, the further south in France one goes, the more fruit and vegetables people eat. For example, in Toulouse, the quantities of fruit and vegetables eaten are both around half as much again per person as in Lille.

Another big difference between France and the United Kingdom is in the way the vegetables are bought and prepared. In any French supermarket or market square, you will see stall upon stall of beautiful, fresh produce, with an enormously rapid turnover. The French usually buy their vegetables fresh every day. And in consequence, they eat a lot less frozen vegetables than people in Britain.

The final difference between the French and the British way with vegetables is in how they're cooked. In France, vegetables are cooked very gently. This exposes them to much less boiling than is the British habit. The French chef may boil or steam them for a short period, and then toss them in olive oil (or butter!). This means that the beans, carrots or spinach are rather more crunchy than the British are used to. But it also means that several of the natural chemicals that the vegetables contain have not been leached out during the cooking process.

So what are these natural products which can be found in vegetables and fruits? A lot of them have been identified, and their properties carefully studied, both by scientists and by the health food industry. But we are going to argue, once again, that it's important not to jump to conclusions. A healthy food which contains a healthy substance doesn't necessarily make the substance healthy on its own. Just because a particular food is associated with protection against a particular disease, we can't assume that a particular extract from that food will necessarily do the same. The arguments are a bit like those we used in the last chapter when we discussed our criticisms of the Diet-heart Model. Just because some food lowers the level of the 'bad' cholesterol it doesn't necessarily mean that the food is going to stop us from having a heart attack. And this is because we have a less than complete view of how good and bad foods operate, or even exactly what causes heart disease. So we can't jump to conclusions.

THE EVIDENCE FOR FRUIT AND VEGETABLES

Much of the evidence in favour of eating more fruit and vegetables comes from the big international studies. Like the Seven Countries Study, these relate heart disease rates, and those of other illnesses, to differences in national diets.

But there are also several studies, such as the Nurses' Health Study, showing the protective effect of vegetables and fruit *within* populations. What the studies show most clearly is that people who eat more vegetables and fruit are at a much lower risk of developing a number of different cancers. The list is long, and includes lung, stomach and colon cancer, and breast and cervical cancer in women. The risk of heart disease is also lower in people with a high intake of fruit and vegetables. For example, Scotland and Northern Ireland have the highest rates of heart disease in the United Kingdom. And in these parts of Britain much less fruit and vegetables are eaten.

People eating more fruit and vegetables also have a lower risk of stroke. And this is probably because they have lower blood pressure levels. And yet another benefit is in protecting the eyes against some of the effects of ageing. Cataracts, common in older people, and age-related degeneration of the retina, are both less common in people who have always eaten a lot of vegetables and fruit.

A final piece of evidence – vegetarians have a lower rate of heart disease than people who eat meat. This is a difficult one, though, because vegetarians may perhaps be leading much healthier lives in general than meat eaters, so this anomaly may possibly be explained by other aspects of their lifestyle.

A HIGH INTAKE OF FRUIT AND VEGETABLES MAY PROTECT AGAINST:

Certain cancers including:

Lung	Larynx	Oral
Stomach	Cervix	Bladder
Breast	Prostate	Large bowel
Pancreas	Oesophagus	

Heart disease

Stroke

High blood pressure

Cataracts

Age-related degeneration of the retina

WHAT ARE THE GOODIES IN FRUIT AND VEGETABLES?

We are going to deal with three possible candidates, two of them briefly and one in much greater detail.

The first candidate is potassium. This is a mineral very much like sodium, the main constituent of table salt. But sodium and potassium seem to have somewhat opposite effects. This may be because in the body they are found on opposite sides of the cell wall, or membrane. And in some cells, like nerves and muscles, leakage of very small amounts of sodium or potassium across the cell wall can make the nerve cell fire off a message, or a muscle cell contract. What this may mean is that a very small change in the amount of sodium or potassium in the diet could have a major effect on the nerves and muscles. And the muscles which may be most affected are not the ones we use to move our arms or legs, but those in the heart or in the walls of the blood vessels.

A lot of potassium in the diet seems to lower the levels of blood pressure. This is particularly true if more potassium is combined with reducing the amount of sodium eaten. And in turn, a lot of potassium in the diet, especially in the form of fruit and vegetables, seems to reduce the risk of stroke. It also seems likely, although it isn't proven, that more potassium in the diet would also cut the rate of heart attack through its effect on blood pressure.

The second way in which fruit and vegetables may influence the risk of heart attacks is due to the amount of fibre. We are going to deal with fibre in a little more detail in Chapter 7. This is because, in spite of what you may have been taught as a child, most of the fibre in our diet does not come from vegetable 'roughage', like the cabbage which we so hated in our school dinners. In the average person's diet, most fibre comes from bread, and to a lesser extent, potatoes.

But it is the third explanation that we're going to go for – that fruit and vegetables contain a lot of antioxidants. Some of these are vitamins that have been given names, like vitamin C (ascorbic acid), or vitamin E. But the food industry is only just beginning to come to terms with the huge range of different antioxidants in all sorts of fruits and vegetables. And many of these have hardly been identified by name, let alone by their properties, either individual or combined.

Let us explain, then, what an antioxidant is. It means a bit more chemistry homework. And going back to the unsaturated, double bonds in the fatty acids that we introduced you to in the last chapter.

UNSATURATED FATTY ACIDS, OXIDATION AND ANTIOXIDANT PROTECTION

If you leave butter for long enough, it will become rancid. This is a very different process from leaving milk to go sour. But both of these processes involve some change in the natural chemicals found in the food.

When milk goes sour, it's because some bacteria in the milk turn the milk sugar, or lactose, into an acid, lactic acid. This is the process used in making yoghurt or cheese. And in fact, in order to make yoghurt in a more consistent and controlled way,

it's possible to introduce the bacteria as a culture into warm milk. But when a fat goes rancid, it's the fatty acids in the fat that are damaged. This happens in the long carbon chains of the fatty acids making up the fat, which we first introduced you to in Chapter 3, and we show again in the diagram on the opposite page. These chains are chemically attacked by oxygen. This must come as a bit of a surprise, because we don't often think of oxygen as doing damage. But a combination of two different circumstances make such an attack possible. One is to do with the fatty acids, and the other with the oxygen itself.

As we saw in Chapter 3, fatty acids may contain one or more unsaturated, or double, bonds. And rather than making the links in the carbon chain stronger, these actually weaken the bond. It is at this point in the chain that the oxygen attacks. The second factor increasing the chances of oxidation is the presence of more highly active oxygen molecules. Among these are ozone, which is like oxygen, but in supercharged form. And there are also other chemicals which have an extra oxygen particle stuck in them, so activating the oxygen in the process. Hydrogen peroxide is one such example. Anyone who has bleached their hair with this chemical would have noticed that it can give off little bubbles of oxygen, during which process the oxygen is very reactive.

When these oxygen particles attack the unsaturated bond in the fatty acid, a series of changes takes place, which eventually cause a break in the fatty acid. And once this chain is broken, the fragments of carbon chain can be released, having had some of the activity from the oxygen particles transferred to them. These new active carbon chains can go on to produce further attack, and damage, on unsaturated bonds in other fatty acids or different bits of the same one. The term 'free radical' is a name given to these very active particles – both the active oxygen itself, and the chemicals that are produced when oxygen causes damage.

OXIDATION OF A POLYUNSATURATED FATTY ACID

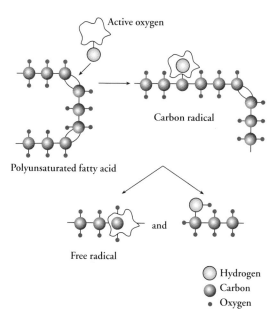

Active oxygen

Carbon radical

Polyunsaturated fatty acid

Free radical

and

○ Hydrogen
◉ Carbon
• Oxygen

Over the last few years we've begun to understand how important this whole process of oxidation is. For instance, the body can actually use these chemicals. By producing reactive oxygen particles, or other highly active chemicals, the body can do things like destroying bacteria which invade the body. So free radicals can do us a great deal of good. But the one area where they can produce damage is in the two major routes to the production of heart disease: atherosclerosis and thrombosis.

FREE RADICALS AND ATHEROSCLEROSIS

In Chapter 1, we described how it is that cholesterol is laid down to produce the thickening and damage to the artery wall which is called atherosclerosis. The first step in that process is that the main cholesterol-containing particles, low-density lipoprotein, gets into the artery wall. There the cholesterol is taken up by cells from the blood stream, and these cells can then coalesce and decay to produce deposits of free cholesterol. What is a major puzzle, though, is

why this only sometimes happens. In some cases cholesterol is taken up by the cells and handled completely normally. But in other instances, the cholesterol is taken up and a foam cell is the result. The answer seems to be, at least in part, free radicals.

As we said in Chapter 3, most of the cholesterol in the blood is carried in a particle called low-density lipoprotein – the 'bad' cholesterol. This particle can become oxidized. When this happens, the free radicals which are produced can alter the shape and structure of this low-density lipoprotein. And then the oxidized low-density lipoprotein is no longer dealt with through normal and healthy breakdown pathways. Instead it is taken up by the blood cells in an abnormal way, and produces the foam cells (see diagram on page 10).

What this may mean is that we have to add a new dimension to our understanding of the role of cholesterol in causing atherosclerosis. Until now, we've imagined that it's simply a high level of cholesterol in low-density lipoprotein particles which increases the risk. And that it's plenty of the high-density lipoprotein particle, which removes the cholesterol from the artery wall, that protects. But we now realize that something else determines the likelihood of producing a foam cell – namely how much damage, through oxidation and free radical mechanisms, has taken place in the low-density lipoprotein particle. And another relevant factor is that oxidation occurs more readily in low-density lipoprotein particles that have a lot of unsaturated, double bonds inside them – in their polyunsaturated fatty acids.

OXIDATION AND BLOOD CLOTTING

It seems, though, that it's not just atherosclerosis which is increased in the presence of the products of oxidation. The cells in the blood which stick together to stop bleeding, for example, after a pin prick, are called platelets. These tend to coalesce after a whole variety of different provocations. One of these is when they are exposed to low-density lipoprotein. But when platelets are exposed to low-density lipoprotein which has become oxidized, they stick together much more enthusiastically. And various other processes in the blood clotting pathway are also stimulated by oxidation of low-density lipoprotein.

We can see, then, that someone who has had a lot of oxidation of their low-density lipoprotein will be at risk of more atherosclerosis, because they will make more foam cells. But because their platelets are more sticky they are also more likely to clot the blood in their narrowed blood vessels to produce a heart attack.

So why doesn't this happen all the time? The answer may lie in the presence of natural chemicals in the body which can protect against oxidation: the antioxidants.

ANTIOXIDANTS – NATURE'S METHOD OF SELF-PROTECTION

A whole variety of chemicals act to protect the body from the damaging effects of attack by oxygen and other free radicals. The first line of self-defence is that most cells in the body have particular enzymes which are capable of mopping up the free radicals. These enzymes, which are chemical catalysts produced by the body, use tiny amounts of metals such as selenium, manganese, zinc or copper to work effectively. The second mechanism of protection lies with a range of naturally occurring antioxidants. Many of these we recognize as essential in our diet.

Perhaps the best known, and certainly the most widely used, is vitamin C, the major vitamin found in fresh fruit and vegetables. Next in line comes vitamin E, which is found in wheat kernels, nuts, corn and safflower oil and olive oil. For a long time this vitamin was without any known function in humans. But it's now seen to be a most important antioxidant. It is, indeed, this property which makes it so popular with the health food industry. There are claims that it can prolong life which, as we will see, may have a grain of truth. But it's also claimed that it can make your skin ten years younger, for which the evidence is, to say the least, questionable!

And apart from these two vitamins, there's a huge variety of other naturally occurring antioxidant chemicals. Some of these act directly as antioxidants, while others, like selenium, are essential in our diet to help the body's antioxidant enzymes. Some naturally occurring antioxidants are:

• beta-carotene and alpha-carotene which are found not only in carrots, as their name suggests, but also in oranges and other yellow and orange fruits and vegetables;
• flavonoids which occur in a wide variety of fruits and vegetables;
• selenium found in fruit, meat and cereals.

The table on the opposite page lists a whole variety of antioxidants, along with their sources in the diet. But it must be stressed that this list is far from complete.

> ### Other vitamins may also defend our arteries
> *It has been suggested that folic acid, found in leafy vegetables, and pyridoxine (vitamin B6), which occurs in meat, fish, cereals and vegetables, may also be good for our arteries. These vitamins help the action of an enzyme which removes from the blood a chemical, called homocysteine, which damages the blood vessel wall.*

TABLE OF ANTIOXIDANTS

Nutrient	Vitamin C	Vitamin E	Vitamin A	Alpha/ Beta-carotene	Selenium	Flavonoids
Other name	Ascorbic acid	Tocopherol	Retinol	Alpha-carotene and Beta-carotene. Carotene may be converted to retinol (vitamin A) in the body.		Flavones (apigenin, luteolin) Flavonols (quercetin, kaempferol, myricetin) Antho-cyanins Catechins Flavanones
Some possible actions	Antioxidant. May reduce certain cancers, ease common cold, fight bleeding. Higher intake associated with higher 'good' (high-density lipoprotein) cholesterol.	Antioxidant. May reduce heart disease by reducing oxidation of 'bad' (low-density lipoprotein) cholesterol, inhibiting platelet activity and preventing blood clots. May reduce risk of cancers and cataracts.	Antioxidant. May lower risk of cancer of lung, stomach, mouth, colon, prostate, breast, cervix. May lower risk of heart disease.		Helps the body produce antioxidant enzymes. May reduce the risk of cancer, inhibit platelet activity and reduce blood clotting.	
Good food sources	Fresh fruit and fruit juices and green leafy vegetables	Vegetable oils, wheat germ, oatmeal, peanut butter, nuts, brown rice	Milk, butter, cheese, egg yolk, liver and some fatty fish	Green vegetables, yellow and red fruits and vegetables	Fish, meat, cereals, little in milk, vegetables and fruit	Vegetables and fruits (especially onions and apples), beverages (tea and wine)

FREE RADICALS AND ANTIOXIDANTS — TYING THEM IN WITH UNSATURATED FATTY ACIDS

These chemical reactions which occur in the body would suggest a simple interpretation: that the more antioxidants in one's diet, the lower the risk of heart disease. In fact, the 'bad', low-density lipoprotein particles contain vitamin E and some other antioxidants. These seem to act to help prevent the low-density lipoprotein particle from becoming oxidized and in turn from damaging the artery wall. And what's more, increasing the amount of vitamin C, and of other antioxidants in the diet, can make

these low-density lipoprotein particles more resistant to oxidation.

But perhaps antioxidants are good not just for heart disease. Some experts think that other changes in the cell caused by free radicals might underlie some of processes which happen in cancer. Indeed, perhaps the clearest example of a cancer-inducing chemical is tobacco. When someone smokes, the burning of tobacco produces vast amounts of free radicals that are inhaled in the form of tobacco smoke. And we know that smoking is the most powerful risk factor not only for lung cancer but also for coronary heart disease.

But it may be a bit more complicated than this.

Smoking and heart disease

People who smoke seem to have much higher levels of damage from oxidation than non-smokers. And this may have something to do with their extra risk of heart disease, as well as cancer. It can be shown that smokers mop up the antioxidant vitamins more than non-smokers. What this might mean is that people who smoke need even more of these antioxidants in their diet. But we must stress that the answer to the health hazards of smoking is not to gobble vitamin C or vitamin E tablets, or even to eat more fruit and vegetables. Stopping smoking has, time and again, been shown to add years to one's life. And by comparison, anything else is incidental.

As we have said, the fatty acids which are most at risk from oxidation are those which have the largest number of unsaturated, double bonds. This could be one interpretation for the margarine studies we mentioned in Chapter 3. And it might mean that a high intake of polyunsaturated fatty acids might actually *increase* the risk of oxidation of a low-density lipoprotein particle. As we've seen, having more polyunsaturated fats instead of saturated fats in the diet lowers levels of low-density lipoprotein cholesterol. But could it be that extra oxidation of low-density lipoprotein might cancel out some, or much, of the benefit of polyunsaturates? This might suggest another reason why substituting polyunsaturated fats for saturated ones in the diet does not necessarily have any benefit in terms of coronary heart disease. And that's in addition to the two possibilities we outlined in the last chapter – that polyunsaturated fatty acids lower levels of the 'good', high-density lipoprotein cholesterol as well as the 'bad', low-density lipoprotein one; and, the

possible harmful effect of the trans fatty acids in hydrogenated vegetable oils.

But in a way, nature has come up with its own solution. If we look at what's the best source of vitamin E, we find it in largest amounts in those things used to make vegetable oils – sunflower seeds and olives, and in the oils themselves. It's as if with every double bond comes its guardian angel standing by.

VITAMIN E CONTENT OF OILS

	MG PER TABLESPOON
WHEATGERM OIL	43
SUNFLOWER OIL	15
SOYA BEAN OIL	10
OLIVE OIL	1.5
MARGARINE	2.5
BUTTER	0.6

Studies show that the diet which most reduces the risk of oxidation of the low-density lipoprotein, as we'll see shortly, is one high in vitamin E and some other antioxidants. But another thing that can be shown to protect against oxidation is a diet high in monounsaturated, and not polyunsaturated, fat. So this provides more evidence for the olive oil argument we outlined in Chapter 3.

THE EVIDENCE FOR ANTIOXIDANTS

Recognizing the importance of free radicals, and the defences against them, as part of the cause of both heart disease and cancer has led to an explosion of interest in antioxidants. Does the evidence hold water? It's certainly looking pretty strong but it must be said that until now, all we can say is that we've got a high index of suspicion rather than 100 per cent proof. Let's give you the evidence and let you decide.

Strong support for the role of antioxidants in preventing heart disease comes from three sources.

Firstly, there are the international comparisons

RELATIONSHIP BETWEEN DEATH RATES FROM CORONARY HEART DISEASE AND VEGETABLE AND FRUIT CONSUMPTION

(——— = estimate of expected rate of heart disease at any level of vegetable or fruit intake)

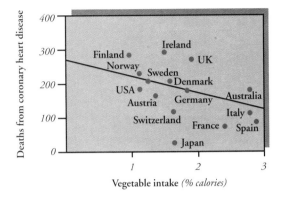

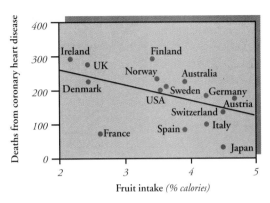

of heart disease rates outlined in the graphs opposite. These show relationships between high death rates from heart attacks and low intake of fruit and vegetables.

But, as we've already said, there are several large differences in the diets of different countries. Fruit and vegetables are just one dimension.

The second piece of evidence comes from studies *within* populations. This approach is to look at how often different sorts of disease develop in people whose usual diet has been studied. And there are three which have shown benefit from antioxidants in the diet. In a report from the Nurses' Health Study, for example, Professor Walter Willett and his colleagues followed more than 87,000 of the American nurses in the study, over a period of eight years, to look at heart disease. They found that those nurses who had the highest intake of vitamin E had only around two-thirds of the risk of heart attacks than those on the lowest intake.

In another study, this group of scientists also showed a similar protective effect for vitamin E in men. And in these men they also found a benefit from carotene. And from the Netherlands came a similar study, in which around 800 men had a detailed diet history. But this time they found a strong protective effect from different antioxidants, flavonoids,

mainly in onions and apples, but also in tea.

The final set of evidence comes not from studies looking at heart attacks or death rates. Instead the approach is to look at possible ways that the antioxidants might work. A huge number of studies of this type have looked at the oxidation, in a test tube, of the low-density lipoprotein particles. And they have shown that supplementing the diet with vitamin E or with flavonoids makes the low-density lipoprotein more resistant to oxidation. What's more, as we've noted earlier, substituting monounsaturated for polyunsaturated fats in the diet can also protect these cholesterol-rich particles from oxidation. And all these mechanisms may have their parallel in the body. In similar fashion, supplementing the diet with vitamin E or flavonoids, or with selenium, makes the platelets less sticky. This may make them less likely to coagulate on the wall of the blood vessel, so causing heart attacks.

If antioxidants are so good, shouldn't we all be taking vitamin E tablets? In other words, should we be popping pills or eating more vitamin E and antioxidants? The definitive answer to this question is, as yet, 'we don't know'.

The result of the Nurses' Health Study might at first support the pill-popping view as the women with the highest vitamin E intake were strongly

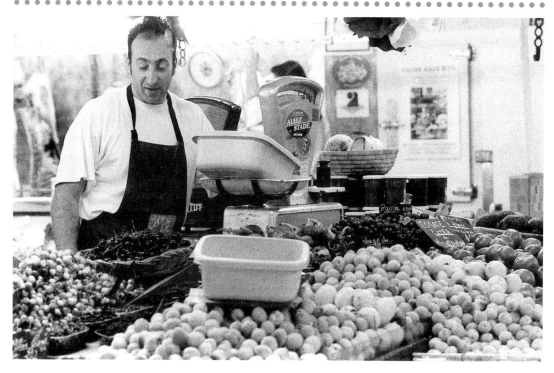

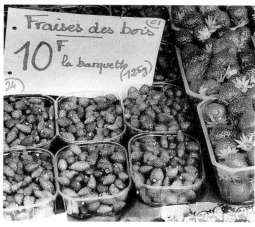

The antioxidants in fruit and vegetables seem to have an important protective effect against heart disease. Even if some studies suggest that vitamin E is more effective in tablet form, a look around French markets suggests that they do not need to rely on tablets for any antioxidant vitamin.

protected from heart disease. But around one in seven women in that study were taking vitamin E as tablets, either alone or as multi-vitamins. And it was in this group, in particular, that the lower rates of heart disease were seen. While it may have been the vitamin E in the supplements which was responsible, these women were also more likely to exercise regularly and less likely to smoke, and per-

haps lead healthier lifestyles in other ways. So the answer is not 100 per cent clear.

Medical scientists generally agree on the best way to find out whether particular interventions produce particular benefits. This is by doing a randomized trial. In these trials, two groups of people, similar in all other respects, are given either vitamin E (or whatever else is under study) or a dummy tablet, known as a placebo. Several such studies are already in progress, looking at whether vitamin E, or alpha-carotene, or beta-carotene, or vitamin C, can prevent heart disease. There is also a possibility that these antioxidants may protect against cancer which is another question being studied. But the trials have not, as yet, provided any clear answers.

In one study in China, supplementing diets with beta-carotene, vitamin E and selenium reduced the risk of cancer. But in a similar study in Finland, vitamin E had no effect, while beta-carotene tablets actually seemed to produce a small increase in cancer risk. Neither study was large enough to give meaningful answers about heart disease.

WHERE DOES THIS LEAVE US? FRUIT AND VEGETABLES OR ANTIOXIDANT SUPPLEMENTS?

Our conclusion is that fruit and vegetables are good news. People who eat plenty of vegetables and fruit are less likely to die at a younger age.

But many questions remain unanswered, including whether it's the fruit and vegetables, or some other aspect of that person's lifestyle. There is pretty good evidence for the benefit of antioxidants in fresh fruit and vegetables, but, as yet, not which one (or ones), or which particular combination. It may be that nature knows best. Perhaps it's the variety of different antioxidants found in most plants which is nature's way of protecting itself against a whole chain of chemical reactions which can do

harm. If this is so, trying to purify any one of the chemicals, to turn into a pill, may be less successful than using nature's entire set of defences against natural forms of attack. But we can bet that over the next few years the food and pharmaceutical industries are going to be searching pretty hard. Natural antioxidants are fast becoming a very saleable commodity to prevent and treat disease.

Fresh fruit is a real pleasure. Tomatoes, in particular, are a treat, and are very rich in all sorts of antioxidants. They may be the best explanation for the low rates of heart disease in France, Italy and the rest of the Mediterranean. An apple is no more expensive than a packet of crisps or a bar of chocolate. But which of us or, especially, which of our children, would grab an apple for a snack, or even think of chewing a carrot! But in that simple substitution, we would be getting less fat, less salt and more antioxidants.

As to vegetables, there is an amazing selection available to most people. And if you take up some of the hints of our cooks, vegetables can provide a most interesting addition to any meal. Do as the French do. Cook them lightly, for example by steaming them, or using the microwave. Toss them in a bit of olive oil, with some seasoning, and maybe some nutmeg. And then, rather than thinking of vegetables as 'eat your greens' or 'roughage', you will discover a whole new dimension to the pleasure of eating. And whether you are doing yourself any good, through potassium, fibre, or antioxidants, you will certainly be improving your *quality* of life.

5

WINE, AND PREFERABLY RED: CANDIDATE 3

'Drink a glass of wine after your soup, and steal a rouble from the doctor.'
RUSSIAN PROVERB

WINE AND THE FRENCH

The French are pretty well known as far as their drinking habits are concerned. Let's look at the figures (see graph below) for a year picked out at random, say 1988. In that year, on average, every man, woman and child in France drank 3 glasses of wine, or shots of alcoholic drink, a day. This compares with a figure of around 2 in the United Kingdom and the United States and only one in Norway. But

AVERAGE ALCOHOLIC INTAKE PER PERSON (1988)

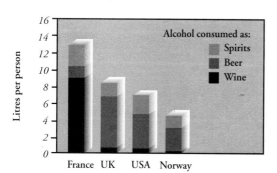

the biggest difference between France and Britain is not so much in how much alcohol is drunk as in the way in which it's drunk.

In 1988 the French were drinking just over 100 bottles of wine a year for each person in the country. This represented, around 70 per cent of all their alcohol. By contrast, the British drank little more than 10 bottles of wine a year, only 15 per cent of all the alcohol consumed. So while the British drink around two-thirds as much total alcohol as the French, in 1988 they were drinking less than one-sixth as much wine.

Habits, of course, are changing. The amount of wine drunk in, for example, Britain has gone up around five-fold over the past twenty-five years. And in France the trend is in the opposite direction. But among all the countries around the world, only four others can get within the same ballpark as the French in their intake of wine. The Italians drink around 87 per cent as much wine per person as the French, the Spanish 71 per cent, the Swiss 64 per cent and the Austrians around 43 per cent. After that, every other country drinks less

AVERAGE ALCOHOL DRUNK AS WINE PER PERSON (1988)

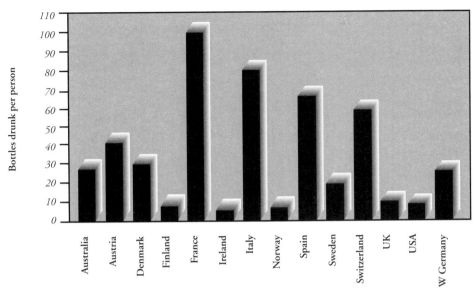

than one-third as much wine as the French.

In this chapter, we're going to look in some detail at the connection between wine and heart disease. We'll pick up on the antioxidant story once again, to show that wine has a lot in it besides alcohol. But there's one other big difference between drinking wine and drinking spirits or beer – apart from what's in the glass.

The French drink while they eat. Wine is an accompaniment to food. The British, who drink mainly beer and spirits, tend to drink without eating, and eat without drinking. And as we will see, there are reasons for thinking that it is not just *what's* in the drink, but *when* we drink it that may make the difference.

IS DRINKING GOOD OR BAD FOR YOU?

Ask an epidemiologist whether alcohol is good for you and they will start talking about U-shaped curves. What's this all about?

This diagram opposite shows what this means. People who drink a large amount of alcohol have a higher risk of dying. This is because they are at risk

GENERAL RELATIONSHIP BETWEEN ALCOHOL CONSUMPTION AND DEATH RATES IN MEN

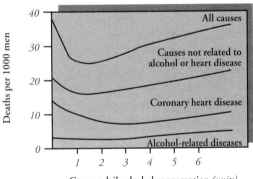

Current daily alcohol consumption *(units)*

from a whole range of problems, including high blood pressure, strokes, cirrhosis and, of course, accidents. In this respect, alcohol is like tobacco – the more you consume, the more dangerous it is. But, unlike cigarettes, the lowest death rates are not seen in the non-drinkers. Instead, we see that lowest risk in moderate drinkers.

The reason for this is that moderate alcohol intake seems to protect against heart attacks. And while most studies find that heavy drinking (six or more units per day – see opposite for explanation of units) is dangerous for other reasons, in only a few is there any suggestion that heavy drinking is a greater risk in heart disease. As a result, most people agree that there's a U-shaped, or even J-shaped, curve for all risks. There may also be one for heart attack risk. But without doubt, the lowest overall risk is in people who are moderate drinkers.

> '*There is no other drug that is so efficient at preventing heart attacks as the moderate intake of alcohol.*'
>
> PROFESSOR SERGE RENAUD, MD, DIRECTOR OF THE FRENCH NATIONAL INSTITUTE OF HEALTH

This immediately raises two important questions. Firstly, why should people who don't drink have a higher risk than people who drink moderately? And, secondly, what do we mean by moderately?

The first thought that goes through someone's mind when confronted with evidence like this is to question whether it's genuine. The U-shaped, or J-shaped, curve has now been described by several different, and very comprehensive, studies, so the results do appear to hold water.

Could it be, then, that people who don't drink might have given up for health reasons, either on their own or on medical advice? We wouldn't lump together as 'non-smokers' both people who have never touched a cigarette in their life with those who have just given up because they had coughed up some blood, or had developed a pain in their chest. If we did, we'd find that these 'non-smokers' were pretty unhealthy, because they included a large number of ex-smokers. And for the same reason, people have looked very carefully at the alcohol story to see whether the higher heart disease risk in non-drinkers can be explained by including ex-drinkers or ex-problem-drinkers. But even lifetime abstainers seem to be more at risk than moderate drinkers.

UK DEPARTMENT OF HEALTH RECOMMENDATIONS ON MAXIMUM ALCOHOL INTAKE

MEN	4 units per day
WOMEN	3 units per day
1 unit equals	½ pint of beer
	1 measure of spirits
	1 glass of wine

Before we go on to question why this might be, let's tackle the question of what we mean by 'moderate'. There's an old medical joke that the definition of an alcoholic is someone who drinks more than their doctor! So there's a risk of doctors defining 'moderate' as 'more than none, but less than one drink'. Different reports have come up with different answers as to how many drinks per day produce an increasing risk of death. Some of these suggest that any more than three drinks a day is risky while others have come up with higher numbers. But what's clear, from more or less every study that has been done, is that the risk of all sorts of other diseases starts increasing dramatically in people who drink more than three or four units a day. What this means is that the guidelines recommended by the UK Department of Health are pretty sensible. These say that men should not drink more than 4 units a day, and women should stay below 3 units a day. And to remind you, one unit of alcohol is half a pint of beer or one measure of spirits. Or, as we will hope to persuade you in this chapter, one glass of wine.

IS IT MODERATE ALCOHOL INTAKE – OR MODERATE WINE DRINKING?

If we look at the comparison of heart disease rates in different countries, we find that the nations where the most alcohol is drunk have the lowest rates of heart disease.

From these studies, it also seems that total death

RELATIONSHIP BETWEEN ALCOHOL, DRUNK AS WINE, BEER AND SPIRITS, CONSUMPTION
AND HEART DISEASE IN MEN (1973)

(——— = estimate of expected rate of heart disease at any level of alcohol)

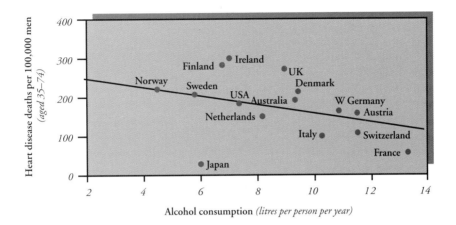

RELATIONSHIP BETWEEN WINE CONSUMPTION ALONE AND HEART DISEASE IN MEN (1973)

(——— = estimate of expected rate of heart disease at any level of wine consumption)

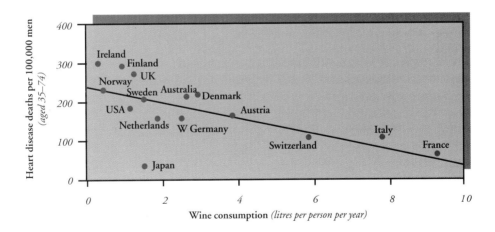

rates tend to be lower in these countries. What this means, in other words, is that people in countries with higher alcohol intake tend to live longer. But when we do these international comparisons, using the amount of wine drunk, rather than the total amount of alcohol, we find that the link with low heart disease rates seems rather stronger.

And it's not only *between* countries that we find these links. Let's go back to have a look at the French. Even *within* France there are regional differences in the way people drink. Alcohol intake is fairly similar in the north and the south, but not what people drink. In Toulouse, the average middle-aged man drinks three or four glasses of

RELATIONSHIP BETWEEN DAIRY FAT INTAKE AND DEATH RATES FROM HEART DISEASE

(—— = estimate of expected rate of heart disease at any level of dairy fat intake)

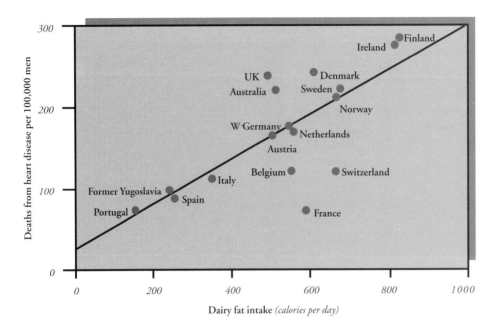

Dairy fat intake *(calories per day)*

RELATIONSHIP BETWEEN COMBINED EFFECTS OF WINE AND DAIRY FAT INTAKE, AND DEATH RATES FROM CORONARY HEART DISEASE

(—— = estimate of expected rate of heart disease at any level of combined dairy fat and wine intake)

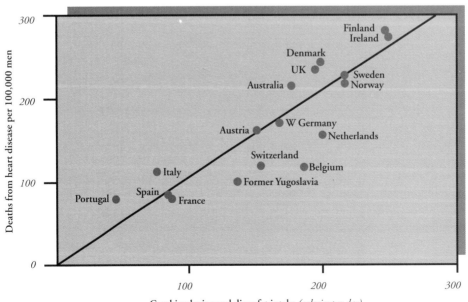

Combined wine and diary fat intake *(calories per day)*

wine a day and virtually no other alcohol. But in Strasbourg near the German border in northern France, people drink only two-thirds as much wine, but rather more beer. And in Strasbourg, heart disease rates are 30 per cent higher than in Toulouse.

But we can hear you muttering that these geographical comparisons can prove almost anything we want them to. Haven't we already used them as evidence in favour of olive oil, against animal fats, and in support of fruit and vegetables? When different people's diets differ so much, how can we tell which difference is the important one?

There are ways that mathematicians can approach this. We show such an approach in the diagrams opposite. The top one shows the relationship between heart disease rates and the amount of dairy fats eaten. And you'll see our old friend, France, having a high fat intake and a low heart disease rate, way off the line. But if, instead, we look at the relationship of heart disease rates with both dairy fat and wine what do we find? Because high wine-drinking nations have low heart disease rates, France is now bang in the place we would expect it to be.

All well and good, but is there any other evidence that wine does any good? What about the big population studies?

One very large study from California looked at heart disease rates in 129,000 people. As in most other studies, the results found the same protective effect of moderate alcohol intake. But their findings also suggested that wine seemed to be more protective than beer, which in turn seemed to provide better protection than drinking spirits. And a most interesting study was recently published from a country which is not usually considered a major wine consumer – Denmark. What these researchers showed in over 13,000 people, followed for up to 12 years, was that drinking around 3 glasses of wine a day reduced the risk of dying from heart disease by some 50 per cent,

while drinking the same amount of alcohol in the form of spirits actually seemed to increase the risk, by around one-third. In this study, beer drinkers seemed to have similar heart disease rates to those of the non-drinkers.

Why, then, does wine-drinking seem to protect the whole French nation if it can't consistently be shown to give the same protection to people living, for instance, in the United States?

Perhaps it's to do with how much wine is drunk. Every day in France, on average, the equivalent of just over one quarter of a bottle of wine, or two glasses, are drunk by every man, woman and child in the country. In Britain and the United States, the corresponding figure is less than one-third of a glass of wine each day.

What this means is that in these countries we might find it very difficult to show any possible benefits from drinking two glasses of wine a day, instead of beer or spirits, just because there are only few people around on whom the figures could be collected.

And what's more, as wine-drinking in the United States and in Britain tends to reflect social status, any differences in heart disease rates may appear to relate to income rather than to drinking habits.

THE STORY SO FAR

To summarize, we have the following pieces of information. Firstly, people who drink moderately have a lower risk of heart disease than people who don't drink at all. Secondly, drinking a lot may put up the risk of heart disease. Thirdly, drinking any more than the UK's Department of Health limits for 'sensible drinking', namely three units a day for women and four units a day for men, brings with it a much higher risk of all sorts of other health problems. And finally, the evidence from international comparisons and from some population studies is pretty suggestive: the benefits of moderate drinking may be greater for wine than for beer or spirits.

HOW DOES ALCOHOL PROTECT AGAINST HEART DISEASE?

People who drink alcohol have higher levels of the 'good', high-density lipoprotein cholesterol than people who don't drink. And this seems to be cause and effect. If someone who doesn't usually drink has their level of high-density lipoprotein cholesterol measured, and then embarks on a period of moderate drinking, the levels will rise, only to fall again when that person stops. All this shows very clearly that moderate levels of drinking increase the amount of the protective cholesterol in the blood stream. And this seems to apply whether the alcohol is drunk as wine, as beer or as spirits. But in contrast, pretty well every study that has looked at the effects of alcohol on the low-density lipoprotein cholesterol has shown absolutely no effect, either good or bad.

> *Understanding high-density lipoprotein*
>
> 'Good', *high-density lipoprotein cholesterol could explain, at least in part, several of the things which we have not previously understood about why particular things are either good or bad for one's heart. As well as moderate drinking, exercise also puts up levels of 'good' cholesterol. And smoking, or having the non-insulin-dependent type of diabetes, gives one lower levels of the protective cholesterol. And in each case, the heart disease risk changes in the opposite direction – down when the high-density lipoprotein cholesterol level goes up, and up when it falls.*

But if we do the sums, it turns out that high-density lipoprotein cholesterol levels can't be the entire answer to why alcohol protects us from heart disease. People with a moderate alcohol intake have around twice as much protection from heart disease as could be explained by their higher levels of the 'good' cholesterol. Put another way, only around half of the protective effect of alcohol seems to come from higher levels of the high-density lipoprotein cholesterol.

What else could it be? Studies indicate that moderate drinking lowers the level of blood pressure and reduces stress. At least some of the remaining benefit is probably because drinking, in moderation, has some effect on the platelets. These are the cells which cause the blood to clot – which is a good thing if one pricks oneself. But, as we've pointed out, it's the blood clot inside the blood vessels, a thrombosis or thrombus, which is the event that precipitates a heart attack. And it seems that a number of things which influence the risk of heart attacks, like alcohol, may do so by their effects on blood clotting – and in particular, by making the platelets less sticky. What's more, moderate drinkers show other favourable changes in blood-clotting mechanisms which may help explain the protection.

WHAT'S SO SPECIAL ABOUT WINE?

Professor Serge Renaud, Director of the French National Institute of Health and Medical Research in Lyon, thinks the solution to the French Paradox is very clear. He feels that the beneficial effects of alcohol are essentially due to the consumption of wine. In Toulouse, he says, the diet is low in butter, and high in bread, vegetables, fruit and vegetable oil. The southern French eat a fair amount of cheese, and foie gras and other very fatty foods are also popular, but all washed down with fairly liberal amounts of red wine. He feels that there are two things going for wine, which differentiate it from other sorts of alcohol: how it is drunk and what is in it.

As we have seen, the differences in alcohol intake between the French and the British are not enormous. But the big difference is in the way that alcohol is drunk. In Britain, some two-thirds of all

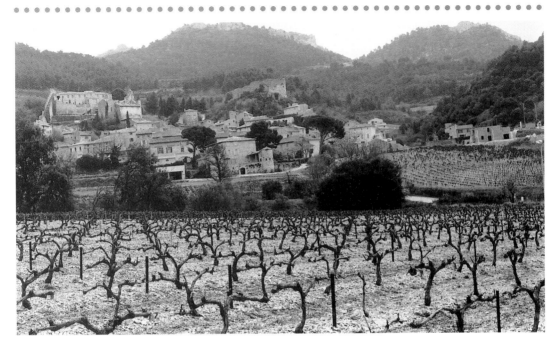

The vineyards of the Côtes du Rhone produce full bodied and strong red wines. Professor Serge Renaud believes that red wine may be the answer to the French Paradox.

alcohol consumed is drunk as beer, and most of this in pubs. And, like spirits, most beer is drunk before or after (or instead of) food. In France, wine is drunk throughout the meal, and it seems that when alcohol is mixed in with the meal, it has a better effect on the levels of the 'good', high-density lipoprotein cholesterol and on the stickiness of platelets than does drinking at other times.

It is, without doubt, also true that binge drinking, and public drunkenness, are much more of a problem in societies where drinking is mainly done separately from eating, and as beer or spirits rather than wine. The 'wine lout' seems less common than the 'lager lout'.

In the last couple of years, there has been a growing interest in the contribution of wine to the explanation of the French Paradox. And a number of scientists have come up with some intriguing observations. The first comes back to the subject of oxidation of low-density lipoprotein, which we introduced in the last chapter. Just to recap, oxidation of low-density lipoprotein makes it even more damaging to the blood vessel wall. This oxidation process also makes the blood-clotting cells, the platelets, more sticky, so increasing the likelihood of blood clots in the vessels to the heart. And we pointed out a number of substances, like vitamin E and beta-carotene, in the table on page 49 which protect the body against such oxidation. And all of these chemicals are naturally present in a whole variety of foods, for example, a range of different fruits and vegetables.

A group of scientists from Davis University in California has found a series of compounds in red wine which are capable of preventing the oxidation of low-density lipoprotein. And it was not only these extracts that were able to prevent oxidation. But red wine itself (in this instance a Californian red!) was more effective in blocking oxidation even than vitamin E. And surprisingly, the wine did so when it was diluted as much as 1000 fold.

The scientists in California found that red wine contained large numbers of the flavonoids, tannins and other natural antioxidants which we mentioned in the last chapter. And as a reminder of the possible benefits of antioxidants – firstly, they block oxidation of low-density lipoprotein – which reduces the leaching of cholesterol into the artery walls. And secondly, by blocking other oxidation pathways, these flavonoids and other compounds reduce the stickiness of the blood platelets.

But it's all very well showing that adding dilute red wine to blood does this or that. More importantly, can the same effect be shown by drinking the stuff? It seems that the answer to that is also yes. A group of scientists from Birmingham University in England forced a group of ten students to eat a meal (presumably free) with half a bottle of wine. They were able to show a marked increase in the blood's defence against oxidation for more than four hours after the meal. And a group of Japanese researchers showed that this protection was given by red wine (Château Lagrange 1989), drunk each day for two weeks, but not by the same amount of alcohol in vodka.

These ideas are all still very new and, as yet, pretty theoretical. We know that there is no such thing as 'proof' in science, but all of this is a very, very long way away even from what scientists think of as proof.

Let's summarize what we do know. We know that oxidation is important both in atherosclerosis and in blood clotting. We think that antioxidants might prevent heart disease. It seems that wine, and especially red wine, contains a lot of antioxidants. And these can both reduce the oxidation of the low-density lipoprotein, and make blood less likely to clot. But we just don't know enough, as yet, to say definitely what, why or how much. Or to say that red wine is definitely better than white in this regard.

One small French study has suggested that three glasses of red wine drunk each day has better effects on the high-density lipoprotein cholesterol level and on blood clotting than the same amount of white wine. But neither this small study, nor chemical analyses of different flavonoids, or other antioxidants, in different wines can possibly act as a basis for concrete advice. And furthermore, while most doctors agree that moderate drinking is good for you, the view that wine is definitely the best for you is certainly not universally held.

Having said that, it's worth mentioning in passing a few of the chemicals which are found in wine and which may have positive effects.

SUBSTANCES FOUND IN WINE WITH BENEFICIAL EFFECTS ON THE HEART

FLAVONOIDS
Flavones
Flavonols – Quercetin
Catechins
PROCYANIDINS
PHYTOALEXINS – Resveratrol
SALICYLIC ACID (aspirin)

We met the flavonoids and flavonols in the last chapter because they are found in large amounts in fruits and vegetables. Quercetins are flavonols which are also found in garlic and onions and have been shown to have anti-cancer effects. Catechins have similar antioxidant properties but are different in structure. Procyanidins are very powerful antioxidants which are found in high concentration in red wine. Phytoalexins are natural antifungal agents which occur on the skin of grapes. Because grape skins are kept longer in the pulp during the manufacture of red wine, there are more of these substances in red wine than in white. One of these phytoalexins, resveratrol, increases the level of the high-density lipoprotein cholesterol as well as making blood platelets less sticky.

And one final curiosity, again from Californian studies, is the observation that wine contains salicylic acid, a substance otherwise known as aspirin. There has been much publicity over the last few years about the protective effect of aspirin when it is taken regularly by patients at risk of heart attacks. This is because of its powerful effect in blocking the sticking of platelets, the blood-clotting cells. And it seems that there's enough salicylic acid, particularly in red wine, for this effect to be found in drinkers. This finding, that there are health-enhancing substances given to us by nature, should not really come as a surprise when we remember that aspirin was originally purified from the bark of a tree – albeit the willow and not the vine.

WHAT DO WE CONCLUDE? WINE WITH YOUR MEALS, AND BE SENSIBLE

It's difficult to find doctors and health educators who will actually carry the flag to encourage drinking, and this is because, wherever you look, when the average alcohol intake goes up, so does the number of excessive alcohol drinkers. If we are going to encourage people to drink, they say, all we will do is produce more alcohol-related diseases, like cirrhosis and strokes, and more accidents. We recognize this fear, and in particular we see the risks of encouraging more drinking by, for example, cutting the taxes on alcohol.

We have less anxieties about talking to people as individuals. What we are saying is 'think wine'. A glass or two of wine with your food enhances the pleasure of eating and the pleasure of drinking. Eating should be an enjoyable, sociable and interactive pastime. An extra half hour at the table, with a glass of wine, is what we are saying – and half an hour less in the pub, with a pint less beer, or one fewer double gin and tonic. This could have advantages for health, and it could make eating more pleasurable. And it could do so without anyone increasing the total amount of alcohol they drink.

6

FISH, AND PREFERABLY OILY
CANDIDATE 4

'"It wasn't the wine," murmured Mr Snodgrass ... "It was the salmon."
(Somehow or other, it never is the wine, in these cases.)'
THE PICKWICK PAPERS, CHAPTER VIII; CHARLES DICKENS

When we were young we were told that eating fish is good for our grey matter. Can it possibly be true that it's also good for our heart? This sounds like a ploy by the Ministry of Agriculture and Fisheries to dump a fish mountain – or is it?

FISH AND THE HEART – THE EVIDENCE

In each chapter so far, we've quoted studies looking at national rates of heart disease. We've then found things in the diet which could go some way towards explaining these differences. Such studies don't exist for fish, or at least not quite in the same way. But heart disease rates in just two populations have made people sit up and think – these being the Japanese and the Greenland Eskimos.

We've already come across the figures for heart disease from Japan. Even though there's been a marked increase in heart disease over the last generation, these are the lowest in the industrialized world, around half the levels of the French.

The traditional Japanese diet is very low in fat – although this is changing with the influx of Western eating habits, and fast food chains, since the Second World War. Like the British, the Japanese are an island nation with a very long tradition of fishing. But the Japanese eat far more fish than the British, and often without cooking it!

There are, of course, many other differences between the Japanese people, and their diet, and those of most other industrialized countries. For this reason, it would be difficult to look at the low heart disease rate in Japan and put it down to this one factor. This is why the Greenland Eskimos are particularly interesting.

The traditional Eskimo diet has always included a lot of fish, and the risk of heart disease is a fraction of that of other Scandinavian people, such as the Danes – who otherwise are much more similar, in most respects, than are the British and the Japanese!

It was this observation, made around fifteen years ago, which led to a new understanding about a particular constituent of our diet, the omega 3 fatty acids.

OMEGA 6 AND OMEGA 3

Omega 3 fatty acids are good for reducing stickiness of the blood. As you may remember from Chapter 3, a fatty acid consists of a long chain of carbon particles joined together. The carbon at one end of the chain, an acid carbon, joins up with glycerol. And when three fatty acids link up with glycerol, this makes a triglyceride fat.

A polyunsaturated fatty acid has in its chain at least two unsaturated, or double, bonds. *Where* they are in the chain is the next question. Let's now go down the far end of the fatty acid away from the acid carbon and the glycerol – maybe sixteen or eighteen carbons distant. If we start at the far end, then call the most distant carbon from the glycerol number one, most unsaturated fatty acids have their first unsaturated bond between carbons number six and seven. Chemists call these fatty acids omega 6 fatty acids.

OMEGA 6 FATTY ACID

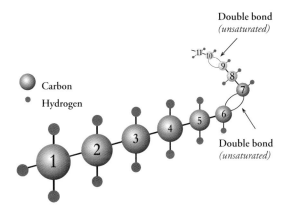

Double bond
(unsaturated)

Carbon

Hydrogen

Double bond
(unsaturated)

But in the green tissues of plants, the commonest polyunsaturated fatty acid has its first double bond just three carbons away from the far end – this being called an omega 3 fatty acid.

OMEGA 3 FATTY ACID

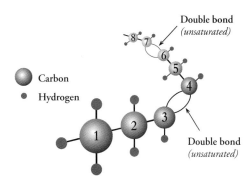

Double bond
(unsaturated)

Carbon

Hydrogen

Double bond
(unsaturated)

Animals which eat green plants include fish, which live on plankton, and cattle. In cattle, most of the omega 3 fatty acid disappears in the bowel, broken down by bacteria. But in fish, and especially oily fish, there are large amounts of omega 3 fatty acids. The most frequent ones are probably the most difficult names in biochemistry – and certainly the most difficult in this book – eicosapentaenoic acid and docosahexaenoic acid.

What do these fatty acids do? They are used by the body in a very similar way to their omega 6 counterparts. They are converted to a variety of different chemicals to make the skeleton of the cells, and are also converted into certain chemical messengers. And one important chemical messenger is the substance vital to the sticking and clumping of platelets which takes place when blood clots. What this means is that platelets work differently in people with a high intake of omega 3 fatty acids. People who eat a lot of oily fish have platelets which are much less liable to clot and stick together than those of people whose polyunsaturated fatty acid intake is largely omega 6.

And this all seems to work out in practice. Platelets from Eskimos show a much lower tendency to stick to a blood vessel wall. And add to this another couple of facts. Firstly, the observation that omega 3 fatty acids, taken as capsules, may reduce levels of low-density lipoprotein cholesterol but not the high-density lipoprotein cholesterol. And, secondly, that they reduce blood clotting by other mechanisms as well. All of a sudden the relative protection of the Eskimos from heart disease seems reasonably understandable.

Which brings us back to olive oil and rapeseed oil and the question of why these might be good for your heart. In Chapter 3 we went into some detail about Professor Serge Renaud's study in Lyon, looking at patients after a heart attack. You may recall that patients were put on a Mediterranean-type diet in which, among other things, saturated fat was largely replaced by rapeseed oil margarine. And this resulted in something like 70 per cent protection against a second heart attack.

In the view of Professor Renaud, this reduction in risk may be something to do with the omega 3 fatty acid content of the rapeseed oil margarine. Although largely monounsaturated, this contains around 5 per cent of another omega 3 fatty acid, called alphalinolenic acid (ALA). In this way the diet may combine the advantages of monounsaturated fatty acids with the benefits of oily fish.

The highest levels of the omega 3 fatty acids are in the oily fish: mackerel, herring, kipper, pilchard, sardine, salmon or trout. Of course, you find fish oil being sold in the health food shops. This is not for vitamins A or D, like for the cod liver oil which used to be recommended for babies and children. It's for the omega 3 fatty acids. In fact, some of the fish oil preparations have names taken from either omega 3 or from the initials of EicosaPentAenoic acid – EPA.

So now we're going to do something a bit different from the previous chapters: having started with the mechanism, we'll see if we can find any evidence. Apart, that is, from the Japanese and the Eskimos.

FISH, OILY OR NOT?

A large study in the Netherlands looked at the risk of heart disease in relation to eating habits over a twenty-year period. The researchers showed that

RELATIONSHIP BETWEEN POSSIBLE RISK OF HEART DISEASE AND AMOUNT OF FISH EATEN

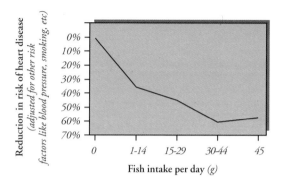

Reduction in risk of heart disease (adjusted for other risk factors like blood pressure, smoking, etc)

0%
10%
20%
30%
40%
50%
60%
70%

0   1-14   15-29   30-44   45

Fish intake per day *(g)*

people who ate fish twice a week or more had around half the rate of heart disease of people who ate no fish at all. What was interesting was that this was not just oily fish but any fish.

This is not the only study to find benefits from fish-eating. In another study, heart disease deaths were reported as strikingly lower in a Japanese fishing village, with a higher fish consumption, than in an inland farming village.

What is perhaps the most interesting piece of evidence about the advantages of fish came from the DART study, in Wales. This was an investigation of some 2000 people who had suffered a heart attack. They agreed to join a study looking at whether one of three different changes in their diet would have any benefit. One group was put on a diet low in animal fat. A second was advised to increase their fibre intake, by having more wheat, oats and other cereal products. A third group was recommended to eat fish twice or more every week. Over the next two years there were 29 per cent less heart attacks, fatal or not, in the group who had been advised about eating fish. But interestingly there were no advantages whatsoever, shown in this study, in cutting back on animal fat or taking more fibre.

One important point to make about the DART study is that it was about preventing a *recurrence* of heart attacks, not the first one. We've already said

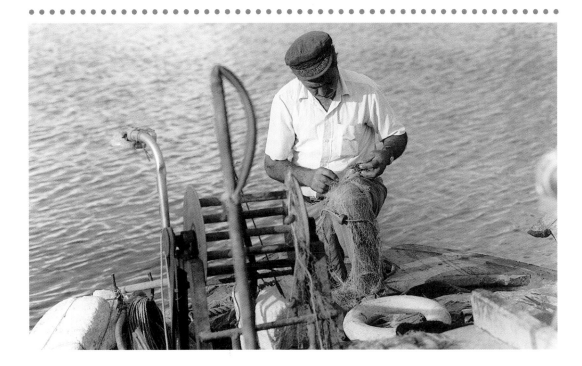

Mediterranean people eat much more fish

than those in northern Europe. Eating

fish regularly seems to reduce the risk of

heart attacks.

that two sorts of damage are necessary before a heart attack happens: the thickening of the wall artery (atherosclerosis) and the clotting of blood inside that damaged artery (thrombosis). If someone has already had one heart attack, we know very well the wall of the arteries to the heart is already thickened and damaged. For this reason, we think that blood clotting plays the main role in influencing who goes on to have a second heart attack. This is why aspirin tablets are particularly useful after a heart attack: they help to stop the blood clotting. The same point may be true about fish and fish oils. So the fact that in these people, eating fish was beneficial, but cutting back on animal fat, or taking more fibre, wasn't, doesn't mean we can all forget

EFFECT OF DIFFERENT DIETS ON THE RELATIVE RISK OF DEATH AND HEART DISEASE (DART STUDY, 1989)

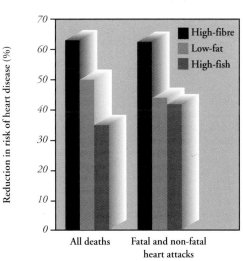

about these last two. In someone with a healthy heart, things could be very different.

But we do seem to have a fair amount of evidence for fish, whether or not people have had previous problems with their heart.

WHAT DO WE CONCLUDE ABOUT FISH?

To summarize, fish is good for you. People who eat fish regularly have fewer heart attacks than non-fish eaters. And after a heart attack, eating fish, and a Mediterranean-style diet – with rapeseed oil – is of benefit. The explanation as to why fish is good for you is probably the fish oils. And in turn, this is probably because omega 3 fatty acids makes blood less sticky. If this is so, the omega 3 fatty acids in rapeseed oil (or soya bean oil) may be just as effec-

tive. We've also seen that omega 3 fatty acids, taken as capsules, have benefits as far as blood stickiness is concerned. But, in the studies we've outlined, any sort of fish is good fish.

So, as for so many other things, we can say with confidence that eating fish is good for you. But as yet, we can't be 100 per cent sure about the same benefits from fish oil extract. Because in some reports, as well as having benefits on reducing blood clotting, these capsules can have harmful effects, for example on blood sugar.

So, back to the theme of the book. It's the belief in healthy lifestyle, not popping pills, that we are preaching. Can fish explain the French paradox? Maybe not. But we'll happily settle down to grilled red mullet, or bouillabaisse, as an answer to the Eskimo paradox.

7

Garlic, Fibre and Salt: Other Possible Candidates

'Wel loved he garleek, onyons, and eek lekes,
and for to drinken strong wyn, reed as blood.'

Canterbury Tales, Prologue; Geoffrey Chaucer

It may seem like this is a chapter of after-thoughts. But there's pretty good evidence that all three of these things are important, and each may have some relevance to the French and their risk of heart disease.

Garlic

Garlic is tasty, as well as healthy. The French have a deserved reputation for liking garlic. And the further south you go in France, the more of it they use. On the Mediterranean a favourite dish is Aïoli – mayonnaise loaded with garlic. This is used to flavour soups, for example, by floating it on croûtons. But some people just eat it on bread. When one of us was a young doctor, he and his wife used to visit a restaurant in London specializing in Mediterranean cooking and where they made a mean Aïoli. On one notable occasion, two days after such a meal, the person in question was given a very sharp verbal rap on the knuckles by an oper-

ating theatre sister: 'If you're going to come into theatres, you shouldn't eat garlic for lunch.' And this was from behind an operating theatre mask!

Garlic has been used for its healing powers for nearly 4000 years. But recently most of the emphasis has been on its effects on the heart.

What can garlic do?

Garlic can reduce the level of the 'bad', low-density lipoprotein cholesterol and increase that of the 'good', high-density lipoprotein – just like olive oil, in fact. It can also make blood less sticky, so less likely to clot. It's also been shown to lower blood pressure, and improve the circulation of blood through the skin. All of these findings have led to a huge explosion in the sale of garlic extracts as a health food in many countries. Indeed, in Germany, garlic preparations are the biggest sellers among all over-the-counter drugs.

So why don't we all start taking garlic tablets?

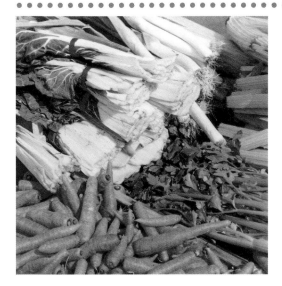

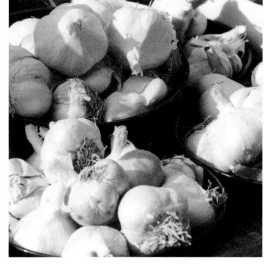

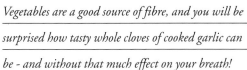

Vegetables are a good source of fibre, and you will be surprised how tasty whole cloves of cooked garlic can be - and without that much effect on your breath!

There are two reasons: one scientific and one social. The main problem with the evidence is that it's not 100 per cent convincing. The trials that have been done with garlic extract, and different preparations of it, have shown very different effects. If you use fresh garlic, instead of the extract, you may have to eat seven or more cloves a day for any real benefit. With this comes the second problem: even if you are behind an operating theatre mask, people will probably be able to tell if you're eating this much! Quite a lot of the garlic preparations give similar problems.

But do experiment with garlic – for its flavour. You'll find garlic in a number of recipes in this book. Crushing a clove on gently cooked vegetables, and tossing them in olive oil, gives a delicious flavour. And one thing we've realized only recently is that if you cook whole cloves of garlic in their skin, and then eat them like onions, they're a very tasty vegetable with a surprisingly mild flavour. Give it a try.

> *'Eat no onions nor garlic, for we are to utter sweet breath.'*
>
> A MIDSUMMER NIGHT'S DREAM, ACT 4, SCENE 2; SHAKESPEARE

FIBRE; NOT JUST WHOLEMEAL BREAD

It's a very strange thing that we have come this far in a book about healthy eating with virtually no mention of the main component of what we eat – fibre. Books about eating for the heart, including this one, talk about reducing fat and meat, and increasing fruit and vegetables, and oily fish. Some, like us, go a little bit off the beaten track, and tell you that wine is a good thing, but otherwise we all say pretty much the same thing. And yet, most cookery books devote the largest part of their recipes to interesting things to do with fish, poultry or meat.

WHAT'S LEFT OUT?

Well, about half of the energy we get from our diets comes from carbohydrates. Some of this is carbohydrate in the form of sugar, either lumps or free-flowing, or in their natural state in fruits and juices. But most of the carbohydrate we eat is starchy carbohydrate. For the British, most of this comes from potatoes and bread, with smaller amounts coming from rice, pasta and breakfast cereals. And there are two separate reasons why these starchy carbohydrates are important in any discussion about healthy eating.

The first is that the more of them one eats, the less one has of other things, such as meat or fat, most of which have a bigger impact on one's heart than the carbohydrate. The second is that almost any form of starchy carbohydrate has with it something called fibre. Let's deal with these points one at a time.

Many scientists believe that the human body is pretty badly designed for the way it now eats. From the days when our evolutionary ancestors first got up on two legs, the human diet was largely one of fruit and grain, with the occasional binge on protein when the hunter-gatherer caught a rabbit or a deer. And from the time we began to settle down to an agricultural way of life, we've eaten a diet that provides something like 75 per cent of its energy intake from carbohydrates and most of the rest from protein, with a little bit of fat. This is the sort of diet that is still eaten across the world, with few exceptions. Most of these exceptions are the industrialized countries of Europe and North America. Here the processing of food, refrigeration and transportation have meant a rapid change in eating habits – at least in evolutionary terms. Only fifty years ago, our diet was predominately carbohydrate. Now it has a much higher fat content overall. We're now eating around 40 per cent of our energy as fats and oils, 15 per cent as protein and only 45

TRENDS IN THE PROPORTION OF DAILY ENERGY INTAKE DERIVED FROM CARBOHYDRATE, FAT AND PROTEIN

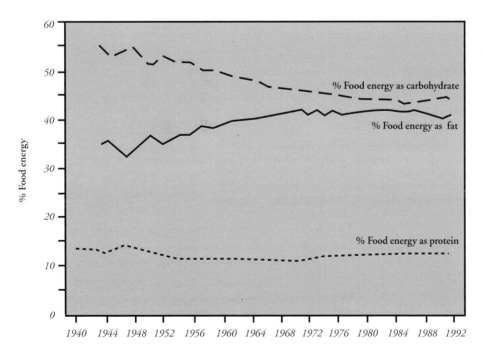

per cent as carbohydrates. This is largely the reason why levels of cholesterol, and particularly the low-density lipoprotein cholesterol, are so much higher in the industrialized countries than in those where a traditional diet is still eaten.

A fascinating study was done by Professor Kerin O'Dea, a nutritionist from Melbourne, Australia. She persuaded thirteen Aboriginal people to return for three months to their traditional lifestyle. This consisted of digging and foraging for roots and vegetables, and hunting kangaroos, birds and other wild animals. During this short period of time, enormous changes were seen in the body chemistry of these people. Their tendency to diabetes disappeared and other risk factors also showed improvements. But we are not writing about an Australian paradox. And far be it from our minds to suggest this as a solution. We just want to use it as a reminder that our bodies were never designed to eat the way many of us do today.

Of all the industrialized nations, Japan beats even France in its low rates of heart disease. Japan is a remarkable country, in that until around a hundred years ago it was completely isolated from any contact with the outside world. And in spite of an influx of fast food chains and burger joints into Japan over the last decade, the Japanese diet is still very low in fat and high in carbohydrate.

DIETARY CHARACTERISTICS OF JAPAN AND THE USA IN THE 1960S

Food	Japan	USA
Fat (% energy)	11	39
Saturated fat (% energy)	3	18
Vegetables (g/day)	198	171
Fruit (g/day)	34	233
Pulses (g/day)	91	1
Breads and cereals (g/day)	481	123
Potatoes (g/day)	65	124
Meat (g/day)	8	273
Fish (g/day)	150	3

When the Seven Countries Study was conducted in the 1960s, only one-tenth of the daily food intake in Japan was from fat, compared to around four times that amount in Western Europe and the United States. By contrast, the Japanese ate very much more rice, and pulses, such as beans. And with that, the levels of cholesterol in Japan run around 40 per cent lower than in Britain – mostly because of low levels of low-density lipoprotein cholesterol.

DIETARY INTAKE OF FAT, CARBOHYDRATE AND PROTEIN IN THE USA AND JAPAN IN THE 1960S

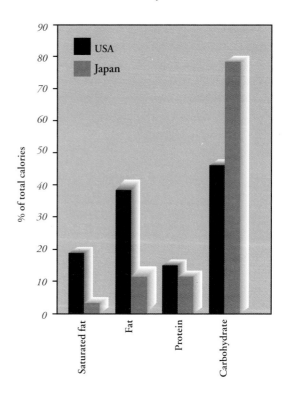

This section is supposed to be about fibre, so where does that come in? The answer is that where there's carbohydrate, there's fibre. Most of the fibre we eat is in bread and potatoes, where most of our carbohydrates come from. But we have a small surprise for you – some fibre is soluble fibre. Shall we try to make ourselves clear?

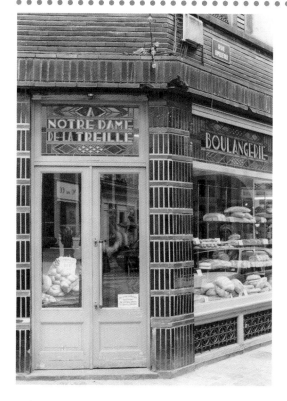

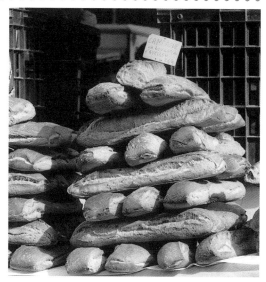

People in France eat a huge amount of bread - before, during and after their meals.

What scientists mean by fibre is carbohydrate which can't be digested and absorbed. If you eat carbohydrate as starch, it is broken down during digestion so that the body can use it. And the breakdown product is a sugar called glucose. But some forms of carbohydrate can't be digested, at least by humans. The cellulose, which cows digest in their intestines with the help of bacteria, is one such carbohydrate which is unabsorbed by humans. But these non-digestible carbohydrates are all fibre – and some of them dissolve in water.

The insoluble fibres are what we usually think of as fibre – wheat bran, wheat-based (or maize-based) breakfast cereals, or wholemeal bread are typical examples. The soluble fibres are largely found in oats, barley and pulses (lentils, peas and beans).

The first of these two, the insoluble fibre, has had a much larger recognition. Dennis Burkitt was a surgeon who went to East Africa some fifty years

ago. He noticed the diseases that he saw there were very different from those he was used to treating in Britain. He very rarely saw people with heart disease. No gall stones. No varicose veins. And he came up with the view that the change in the diet that people in the UK had experienced, compared with what our ancestors in the African plains used to eat, was the explanation for the diseases of Western civilization – including not only heart disease but also diabetes, bowel cancer and gall bladder disease. The logic of his argument was that, by refining our diet, our bowels had nothing to contract on – no roughage – because all the fibre had been taken out. And some thirty years on, since he first published these ideas, there is still a strong belief that he was right, especially as far as bowel disease is concerned. It may well be that a highly refined diet, containing little fibre, just doesn't allow the bowel to work properly in propelling its contents. And this means that the wall of the bowel is exposed to all sorts of toxins, which may increase the risk of cancer, as well as producing constipation and gall bladder disease. But heart disease too?

If any fibre is valuable in preventing heart disease, it is soluble fibre. Several studies have now shown that a diet high in soluble fibre, including oats and pulses, can lower the level of low-density lipoprotein cholesterol. But whether this, in turn, is associated with less heart disease is not at all clear.

One thing we mustn't forget about fibre and carbohydrate is its importance in filling us up. If you try eating three rounds of sandwiches made of stoneground wholemeal bread, you'll see what we mean. Eating fibre-rich food not only fills our stomach more effectively, but our stomach also empties at a more leisurely pace. That heavy feeling under our ribs four hours after a bowl of porridge means that we might not need a bag of crisps in the middle of the morning. And by making us feel fuller, and for longer, this may help explain why high carbohydrate diets are linked with less obesity than we see in most parts of the Western world.

But this leaves an important question, especially in the context of this book. What do the French do about carbohydrate and fibre?

THE FRENCH AT TABLE: WHAT CARBOHYDRATE? HOW MUCH FIBRE?

The traditional entrée at a French meal – in most restaurants and many homes – is just a meat dish, or fish, or poultry, perhaps cooked with a few vegetables. If, in the restaurant, you asked for some potatoes, vegetables or a salad, you would be served this after your main course. But what the French eat in vast amounts is bread. The baguette, with more crust than bread, is chopped up in a small basket or bowl, on the table, and eaten right the way through the meal.

In the restaurant, it's eaten while you wait to order, while your food is being cooked, with the soup or starter, and all the way through the entrée to mop up the sauces. And then, at the end of the

meal, there's the bread and cheese. As a result, the French diet is much higher in fibre than the British – and largely from eating bread rather than from potatoes, rice or pasta (see graph below).

All around the Mediterranean, fibre intake is high. But in some countries it's from bread, in others it's from pasta, potatoes or other fibre-rich vegetables. In Britain, perhaps the most dramatic change in the population's food supply in the last ten years is in the range of bread available. When people thought that fibre just meant wholemeal bread, this loaf had an aura of 'goodness' about it. But go into any bakery or supermarket now, and you'll be spoilt for choice: ciabatta, baked with olive oil from Italy, perhaps even with olives or sun-dried tomatoes; Spanish pan gallego, with whole seeds of wheat and sunflower; a variety of white and wholegrain breads from France; and an enormous selection of really tasty British bread. This huge choice is worth experimenting with, and not just for toast for breakfast, or for sandwiches. Try, as a snack, a ciabatta roll or a slice of toasted three-grain bread with a small drizzle of extra virgin olive oil. And you might even have a go at putting some really fresh bread on the table to eat through your meal. Doing it the French way!

SOURCES OF FIBRE IN THE AVERAGE BRITISH AND FRENCH DIET

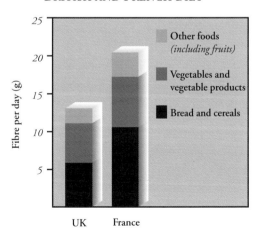

Salt

We don't really think that the French Paradox has much to do with salt, but we'll mention it nonetheless. Some of the salt we eat is sprinkled on during our meal, or added during cooking. But a huge amount of the salt in our diet is used in the processing of foods. So almost every savoury snack we eat, be it crisps or cheese, or biscuits, contains a large amount of salt.

The real name for salt is sodium chloride. But what matters is the sodium. The food industry adds sodium to a lot of things as sodium glutamate, which is what you find in stock cubes and a lot in Chinese take-away cooking. And this is another reason why savoury snacks are rich in sodium, even though it's not, strictly speaking, salt.

So what's wrong with sodium?

Mainly, it's to do with blood pressure. In Chapter 4 we talked about the benefits of fruit and vegetables in lowering blood pressure and cutting the risk of strokes. We said then that fruit contains a lot of potassium, which could explain this. What seems clear is that replacing salt (or sodium) with potassium does lower blood pressure; much more so than just cutting down on salt.

So our message is clear, even though it may not have all that much to do with the French Paradox. Cut back on savoury snacks. If you want a nibble, have some fruit. This will not only exchange sodium for potassium, it will mean that you're eating less fat, maybe less trans fatty acids, more fibre and more potassium.

Conclusion

So there you have it. Loads of theory, lots of recommendations, and all pretty indigestible! And so what we'll try to do is to finish this part of the book by putting it all together: a new 'Diet-heart Model', and advice for a healthy lifestyle, not just a healthy diet.

8

FINALLY, A HEALTHY LIFESTYLE NOT JUST A HEALTHY DIET

'Eat and drink measurely, and defy the mediciners.'
Proverb

Let's start by trying to put together a summary of the ideas we have been discussing. We have set up the Aunt Sally of the old Diet-heart Model; here it is to remind you.

Animal fat ➤ Blood cholesterol ➤ Heart attacks

We have said that we are unhappy with it for lots of reasons – to do with the fact that heart disease is not caused only by cholesterol; blood cholesterol level is not determined solely by animal fat intake; and animal fat may do bad things besides raise cholesterol.

What we've put up instead is a more detailed version of the Diet-heart Model. And we think that this one explains quite a lot that the old one does not. This figure makes the point that atherosclerosis is still pretty central to being the cause of heart attacks. It is what we call necessary but not sufficient on its own. As well as damage to the artery, a blood clot is necessary for a heart attack to occur. The model makes the point that it is only one sort of cholesterol that is responsible for atherosclerosis: the low-density lipoprotein or 'bad' cholesterol. And the process that makes this low-density lipoprotein really dangerous is oxidation. The 'good' cholesterol, or high-density lipoprotein, helps remove deposits from the artery wall, and this protects from atherosclerosis.

The model goes on to make several points. Firstly, a lot of things affect the process of atherosclerosis, besides what we eat. Among the most important are smoking, high blood pressure and diabetes. But there are many others – at the last count over 300 different things had been identified which increase the risk of heart attacks, largely through atherosclerosis! We'll come back to the vital role of smoking – or at least not smoking!

All around the model we've put little arrows to

THE NEW HEART-DIET MODEL

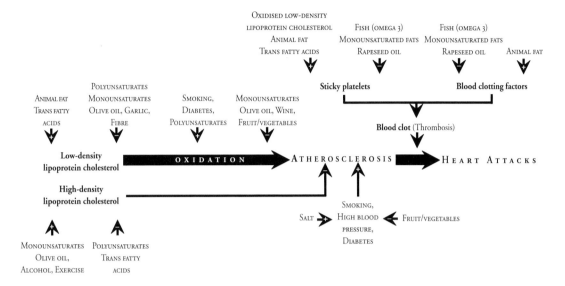

show how these processes can be affected by what we eat. And you'll see that what we eat has an impact at many different stages of the process. Some things put up levels of the low-density lipoprotein cholesterol while others lower these levels. Other factors operate in the opposite direction, by influencing levels of the protective, high-density lipoprotein cholesterol. And we can see that some items are represented on both sides of the equation – sometimes working in the same direction and sometimes opposite. So polyunsaturated fatty acids in the diet, in corn oil or soft margarines, drop the levels of both the 'good' and the 'bad' cholesterol, perhaps cancelling out any benefit. Trans fatty acids get into the diet largely from the processing (hydrogenation) of vegetable oils to make margarines (especially the hard ones), shortening, and some cooking oils. These increase levels of 'bad' and lower levels of 'good' cholesterol, the two effects working in parallel for a bad effect on atherosclerosis. Monounsaturated fatty acids, on the other hand, lower the levels of low-density lipoprotein cholesterol and raise those of high-density lipoprotein cholesterol – both for the good. Other things

in the diet may be of benefit by reducing levels of low-density lipoprotein cholesterol alone (garlic and fibre), or by raising those of the protective high-density lipoprotein cholesterol (exercise and alcohol).

The two main differences of our model from the old Diet-heart Model are the emphasis on both oxidation and blood clotting (thrombosis) in the process. Oxidation is a process that occurs in the body all the time. But it's commoner in smokers, and indeed in people with diabetes. And the diet plays a part in two ways: susceptibility to oxidation, and protection from oxidation. Polyunsaturates increase the amount of oxidation, which may cancel out any benefit they may have in reducing the levels of low-density lipoprotein cholesterol. But quite a lot of the French Paradox is about protection against oxidation. We've shown that there are antioxidants in wine, fruit and vegetables, which may play a large part in explaining the French Paradox. But also, monounsaturated fatty acids are less likely than others to be oxidized. Which may help to explain some of their benefits.

On the blood-clotting side, the most likely

benefits of fish come from their high content of the omega 3 fatty acids. These make the whole process of blood clotting less likely to happen. By working in the other direction, animal fats, oxidized low-density lipoprotein, and trans fatty acids all seem to increase this process of sticky platelets.

There are probably also many influences of what we eat on many of the other things which damage the blood vessel walls. But we're going to limit ourselves to the blood pressure story. We have given you some evidence that salt in the diet tends to raise our blood pressure. And potassium, found in particular in fruit and vegetables, has the opposite effect.

So that's where we'll leave our model for now. And, like everything else in science, this is not the ultimate answer to the ultimate question. It's only in *The Hitch-Hiker's Guide to the Galaxy* that one can get the ultimate answer: 42! But, as you may remember, nobody was sure of the question. Here, we know the question and we can have a stab at the answer. But the ultimate truth will change, as more and more things are discovered which better explain the observations.

A HEALTHY DIET IS PART OF A HEALTHY LIFESTYLE

What we would like to do is to translate the messages of the French Paradox. We are going to propose a set of ten commandments for healthy living. And because healthy living is not just about what we eat, we'll talk about other things that are important as well. We're also going to try to put these commandments into some sort of order.

1 *Avoid smoking at all costs.* You might be surprised to find this at the top of the list in a book about diet. But we've calculated that smoking is by far and away the biggest risk factor – and not just for heart disease. People who smoke have over twice the risk of dying from heart attacks as non-smokers – regardless of whether they eat fish, or butter, or vit-

amin E, or whatever. We've already mentioned, in Chapter 1, that if you're a 45-year-old man, you have around 7½ years less to live if you smoke than if you're a non-smoker. This means that smoking is around twice as dangerous as having high blood pressure and three times as dangerous as having a high level of low-density lipoprotein cholesterol.

EFFECT OF SMOKING ON THE LIFE EXPECTANCY OF A 45-YEAR-OLD MAN

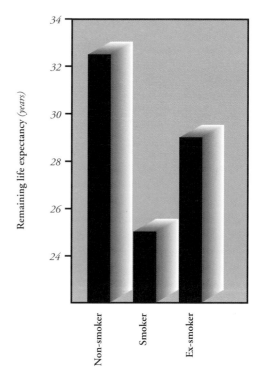

And there's no point in just shrugging this off – giving up smoking is much better at reversing that risk than anything else we can do.

2 *Take some physical activity on a regular basis.* Even spending twenty minutes doing some gentle walking is better than nothing at all. You could try swimming, or getting a bike, or a dog. It doesn't have to hurt to be healthy. Regular exercise improves the circulation. It helps to cut down blood pressure and puts up levels of high-density lipoprotein cholesterol. It also seems to make the blood less sticky and reduce the tendency towards diabetes.

3 *Enjoy your meals in leisurely fashion* and, where possible, not alone. The traditional French meal is a very relaxed affair. And it may well be that this does more than preventing indigestion. It may also reduce some of the more dangerous swings in the chemistry of the blood that happen when food is bolted. In addition, reducing stress and being sociable are probably good for one's heart as well as one's mind.

4 *Vary your food intake* so that eating is more enjoyable. Don't imagine that every day must be similar. Equally, changing the balance of your diet may mean that the chocolate éclair, or the Quarter Pounder with Cheese, is a once-a-month indulgence instead of twice-a-week.

5 *Try to cut back on the amount of fat in your diet* – especially animal fat. There are lots of easy ways to do this without making it a real hassle:

• do less deep-frying;
• have things grilled instead;
• buy lean cuts of meat;
• trim off the obvious fat;
• try semi-skimmed milk;
• cut back on the savoury snacks between meals;
• if you fancy a nibble have an apple, or a carrot, or even a ciabatta roll.

6 *Eat more starchy carbohydrate.* Remember that bread is thoroughly healthy. Put some on the table with your meals, and use it to mop up gravy, just like the French do. Plenty of potatoes, rice or pasta is a better way of filling up than that second helping of meat. And in exchange for the extra carbohydrate, use less fat. Cut back a bit on chips. Spread your butter or margarine more thinly. Or use a low fat spread.

7 *Try using monounsaturated fats* – olive oil or rapeseed oil – for salads or for cooking. And try olive oil or rapeseed oil spreads instead of butter or polyunsaturates. Try a little drizzle of extra virgin olive oil on your toast instead of butter. And remember that we're suggesting that you cut back on the amount of oil used – so this will cancel out some of the extra costs of olive oil.

8 *Eat plenty of fresh fruit and vegetables*, and don't overcook them.

9 *Enjoy a glass or two of wine* with your meals.

10 *Have fish instead of meat*, a couple of times a week.

AND WHAT DO THE OTHER EXPERTS SAY?

Now that we have given our commandments let's look to see how they square up with the previous advice of the experts.

In the autumn of 1994, a new report was produced by a British Government committee, the Committee on Medical Aspects of Food Policy. They produced lots of recommendations about how many slices of bread, and how many potatoes, we should be eating each week. In general, their conclusions were pretty close to our own – although they didn't mention wine or olive oil. They suggested more fruit and vegetables, more bread and potatoes, more fish and fewer dairy products.

But we think it's quite difficult to get one's head around advice like to have four and a half slices of bread a day, three egg-sized potatoes, or four portions of vegetables and two pieces of fruit a day. For many of us, one day is very different from another day. And in our view, it's easier to think of balancing the overall diet, rather than trying to count up the potatoes.

One approach which we've found interesting is something developed in the United States by the

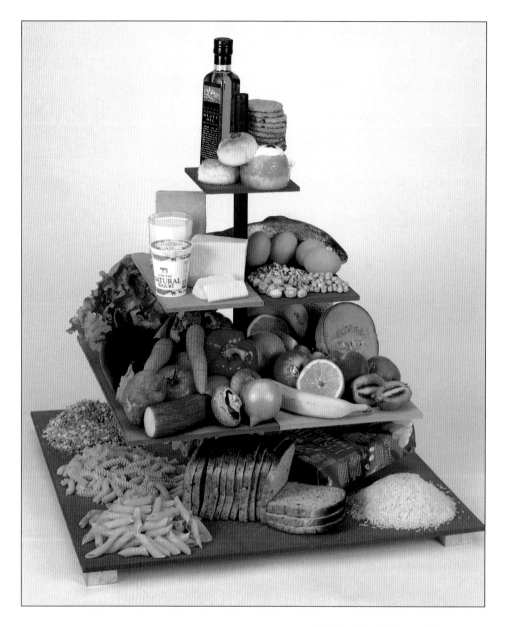

A daily Food Guide Pyramid.

Department of Agriculture. They've put out the idea of a Food Guide Pyramid. What this does is to give a sense of the sort of proportions of different types of food which make a healthy choice, and these foods are grouped into a number of cate-

gories. Like a real pyramid, the whole thing is solidly balanced on a very broad base, which is the starchy carbohydrates. The top of the pyramid is much narrower and consists of small amounts of the fatty foods. These, of course, should be used more sparingly, to avoid toppling the pyramid over. In the middle are various amounts of fruit and vegetables and the protein-rich foods like meat, poultry and fish.

THE DAILY FOOD GUIDE PYRAMID

What the pyramid idea does very usefully is to suggest what is healthy in terms of the amounts of one sort of food versus another. So, a good diet will have more helpings of starchy carbohydrate than of meat, fish or eggs. And this avoids the pyramid being too top heavy. But what the pyramid idea doesn't help us with is in the question of what sort of oil or fat to use (as opposed to meat). And it doesn't even mention wine!

Now you can get on to enjoying the wine and recipes. The rest of this book is about cooking, eating and drinking. It's about making enjoyable snacks and meals using healthy ingredients. We've done what we can to recognize the problems of cost. But remember that a bottle of olive oil costs about the same as a cheap bottle of wine – and lasts much longer.

You'll notice that in the recipe section, we give an estimated breakdown of what's in the recipes. We show the number of calories, then the percentage breakdown of fat, protein and carbohydrate. We also give the percentage of a person's recommended daily intake of the antioxidant vitamins provided by one serving of the dish.

But there are two words of caution. Firstly, what's in a recipe usually differs from what's in a meal because you don't eat just the one course in the meal. Not only will you have something before, and perhaps after, but you will also probably have vegetables, bread and wine. For this reason, we have analysed each recipe as a complete course, or meal, with suggested accompaniments (although the wine suggested to go with your meal has not been included in the analyses). Of course it would be impossible for each meal to meet all the dietary recommendations. While it is important to aim for a diet which is not too calorific, has less than 35 per cent of calories coming from fat, and 100 per cent of the daily intake of the antioxidant vitamins, we recognize that variety is the spice of life. The nutritive value of any diet depends on the overall mixture of foods eaten over the course of weeks, months or years. So we have included some recipes which do not conform as well to the guidelines as others, but the nutritional analyses should help you to maintain a healthy balance.

And secondly, even if we can give you the figures for carbohydrate, for protein and for fat – even saturated, monounsaturated and polyunsaturated – the amounts of the antioxidant vitamins, A, E and C – there's a lot we can't provide. We don't know, for example, which antioxidants may turn out to be the most important in the vegetables, or in the wine. And we won't be telling you about potassium, different sorts of fibres, and so on either.

But this may be no bad thing. We approached this exercise to get across one main message: that eating and drinking can be fun, as well as being healthy. The last thing we want is to make it a new exercise of do's and don'ts. So sit yourself down, fill your glass, and enjoy.

9

WINE, AND PREFERABLY RED – THE CHOICES

by Malcolm Gluck

It comes as a bit of a shock to a man to discover that for two-thirds of his life he's been on a diet. But in the course of thinking about this chapter it struck me, rather forcibly, that I've been on a diet since I discovered French food and French wine some thirty years ago. It was in France that I first happened upon vegetables which actually tasted of something; fish which was alive with flavour; meat, poultry and game of such richness that these beasts were surely unknown in the isles of Britain. Until the early 1960s vegetables had been, for me, rather repellent accompaniments to overcooked pieces of meat, soggy bits of fish and other conglomerations which passed by the name of 'cuisine' in those days. There was little sunshine to excite the blandness of the food, due largely to the spectre of rationing still haunting the dark larder. Foreign holidays, later to expand the gastronomic horizons of millions, were unknown except to the well-off or the eccentric.

It was only in November 1960, when Elizabeth David first published her monumental book *French Provincial Cooking*, that the first heady rays of the southern sun began to light our kitchens. By February 1963, with the fourth imprint of the *vade*

mecum on its way into bookshops, the food revolution in Britain had begun to gain significant pace – and garlic (yes ... as I live and breathe ... garlic!) became more widely distributed than merely in the odd exotic greengrocer's shop.

For the last three decades, then, my regular forms of sustenance, apart from fresh fruit, have been those which are generously laced with olive oil and garlic, and these simple though magical ingredients have insinuated themselves into vegetables, fish, meat, cheese and various breads. I didn't know it when I started it but this appears to be what is now called the Mediterranean Diet. Does it work?

Well, I didn't know, until recently, that the Mediterranean Diet had a putative side effect other than that of providing extreme pleasure; but if looking years younger than you really are and feeling energetic are part of it then this Diet, as far as this body is concerned, is working wonderfully. I'll report back when I reach a hundred and I'm hauled off the tennis court (or chased out of the bedroom by a jealous husband) to receive Her Majesty's telegram. The crazy thing is, of course, that all I do is eat those things I love to eat and drink those wines I love to drink.

These wines are also the wines which go most harmoniously with the kinds of food discussed in this book. That is to say red wines rich in the phenolic compounds bequeathed to them during their maceration and fermentation processes. These compounds can come from the skins but also, in some wines, from the pips and the stalks. They give red wine its colour; they also provide its tannin which is the substance, along with acidity, which red wine needs to slip smoothly into a rich dotage. In white wine, these phenolics play little part and in some cases none whatsoever.

What are these red wines? Well, if you look at the wines that the good people in the south-west of France drink, then these are the red wines of Cahors, wines from the Languedoc-Roussillon (especially Corbières and Fitou), wines from Bergerac and Gaillac and, of course, wines from the northern Rhône (Côtes Rôtie, St-Joseph, Crozes Hermitage and Cornas) and the southern Rhône (of which my favourites, and those richest in flavour, are Châteauneuf-du-Pape, Gigondas, Lirac, Vacqueyras, Rasteau, and Beaumes-de-Venise – not the famous sweet white from this village but the lesser known red). Arguably the richest in tannins, however, are those *vins des pays* made from the tannat grape in the Basque country in deep southern-western France, in the shadow of the Pyrenees, and those usually available include Madiran, Côtes de St Mont, Irouléguy and Tursan. For my part, I would also add to this list the reds of the Loire, called Chinon and Bourgueil and made exclusively from the cabernet franc grape, and the wines of Provence (particularly Bandol with its rich mourvèdre grape constituent). Wine from the specific vineyard called Mas de Daumas Gassac, labelled no more augustly than *Vin de Pays de l'Hérault*, is an especially high-flying elixir though it is equally steep in price. Also excellent are many of the wines from the less well-trumpeted regions of Bordeaux: Fronsac, Blaye and the Premières Côtes. If all these red wines can be said to flaunt one overwhelming

characteristic, it is a savouriness tempered by a fruity earthiness which is richly redolent of herbs and sunshine. They are wines which suit good living and the partnership of well-flavoured foods. The best of them have a thought-provoking complexity.

These characteristics can also be found in certain Italian, Spanish and Portuguese reds. Barolo, Barbaresco, Aglianico del Vulture, some Chianti Classicos and Copertino, for example, from Italy. Priorato, Reserva Rioja, Ribero del Duero, Costers del Segre (look for the name Raimat), and tempranillos or cabernet/tempranillo blends from Penedès (like Torres Gran Coronas) and Valdepeñas in Spain. In Portugal, young reds from the Alentejo and Ribatejo regions are good chilled to drink with fish dishes, but the richest in tannins are the Garrafeira wines using the touriga nacional grape. Wines from eastern Europe can also be tasty: aged pinot noirs from Romania, cabernet sauvignons from Bulgaria, kekfrancos from Hungary (this is also good chilled with fish dishes especially those oily varieties like salmon and mackerel).

Wines made from deeply flavoursome grapes given to basking in sunshine – and sun is crucial to encourage berries to develop phenolic compounds – in countries on the edge of Europe are also good drinking. Some reds from Morocco are ripely endowed with flavour. There is also Château Musar from the Lebanon. But in this age of New World wine there are many wonderful red wines from newer countries which fit our bill of fare. These include the merlots, cabernet sauvignons and pinot noirs of Oregon and Washington State, the zinfandels of California (those made by Ridge vineyards are particularly dazzling and tannin-rich), the cabernet sauvignons of Mexico (look for the name L. A. Cetto) and Argentina (Weinert and Trapiche are good producers), the merlots and cabernet sauvignons of Chile (Caliterra, Concha y Toro and Santas Rita and Carolina) and even, would you believe, the tannat grape variety wines from Uruguay of which the odd bottle is now popping up on British wine shelves. South Africa has its great pinotage wines, pinotage being a much underrated grape which came about by crossing the cinsaut with pinot noir. This country also turns out some wonderfully flavoursome cabernet sauvignons and merlots. A particular estate to note here is Kanonkop, especially its pinotage. Backsberg can also be extremely fine.

Australia, of course, is overflowing with great, rich reds. Among the best are the cabernet sauvignons from Western Australia, the Shiraz and cabernet sauvignons from the Barossa Valley, Clare Valley cabernet sauvignons and merlot blends, Coonawarra cabernet sauvignons, and the reds from the Hunter Valley, Victoria, and the Mudgee (and, in fact, just about everywhere else in the grand island). The great red wines of the Penfolds company, particularly the astronomically expensive Grange Hermitage, are so rich in tannins that you can, should you possess the patience to wait the twenty years necessary to let them precipitate out,

eat them with a spoon. It's always a sign of conscientious wine-making, and usually lovingly grown grapes, when a label encouragingly proclaims that the contents of the bottle will throw a sediment. New Zealand merlots are somewhat rarer, but those bottles with a couple of years of age can be marvellous – if you can find them. The 1994 vintage merlots from New Zealand, many examples of which I tasted in barrel in early 1995, promise to be particularly suited to matching the recipes in this book.

We have so many wines available to us today. Britain, alone, is supplied with wines from nigh on fifty other countries. The choice is vast and even shortening my focus and limiting this section to red wines only has provided a fairly lengthy list. (Or should I say a big, healthy one?) You will see that I have recommended wines to go with the recipes which follow. You may also notice that I have often suggested white wines, too, as it seems that any wine, whatever its colour, could be better for you than no wine at all!

FOR THE RECIPES

Our five cooks have provided recipes using the basic ingredients of a Mediterranean diet – wine, bread, olive oil, fish, garlic, fresh vegetables and fruit – and we have included a breakdown of the nutrients and calorie totals for each of these. However, we do not intend for these to be used to 'calorie count', they are helpful simply to gain an overview of a day's nutritional intake. Although some of the main dishes contain more than the recommended daily intake of 35% calories from fat, if they are eaten as part of a healthy balanced diet much of what we eat in the rest of a week – breakfast cereals, toast, sandwiches and fruit – has enough carbohydrate and relatively little fat, and thus maintains a healthy balance.

Remember it is the diet as a whole and the food and drink you consume over a period of time that is important, and it is the variety in that diet which ensures a

nutritional balance. As we have stressed throughout this book, food and wine are sources of pleasure, and when consumed sensibly will benefit your health and enrich your life. We hope that these recipes help you put into practice some of the lessons we are learning from the French about eating for a healthier heart.

The nutritional information presents the percentage content of fat, protein carbohydrate and vitamins in one serving. (Vitamins are expressed as a percentage of the estimated daily requirement for an adult male, which is 25 mg of vitamin C, 5 µg of vitamin E and 500 µg retinol equivalents from vitamin A and carotene. The symbol '> 100%' indicates that the recipe provides more than the recommended intake of that particular vitamin.) Obviously people differ in the amounts of nutrients and energy (calories) they require, but as a general guide an adult man requires about 2500 calories per day and an adult woman requires about 2000.

Soups

· ·

VICHYSSOISE

Cold Leek and Potato Soup

MIREILLE JOHNSTON

SERVES 4

Leek is one of the most popular vegetables in France, along with the potato. *Vichyssoise* soup is, in fact, not a French invention – French soups are always served warm or hot. Many believe it was created by an American chef. However, this celebrated recipe is based on the traditional French leek and potato soup and is served cold, enriched with a little cream.

50 g (2 oz) butter
225 g (8 oz) potatoes, chopped
4 leeks, white parts only, sliced
2 shallots, coarsely chopped
1.2 litres (2 pints) chicken stock or water

300 ml (10 fl oz) single cream
salt and freshly ground black or
white pepper
2 tablespoons snipped fresh chives or chervil

Heat the butter in a large pan and sauté the potatoes, leeks and shallots for about 5 minutes. Meanwhile, heat the stock or water in a separate pan. Add the stock to the vegetables, bring to the boil and simmer over a high heat, uncovered, for 30 minutes.

Purée the soup in a food processor then pour into a bowl. Stir in the cream and season to taste with salt and pepper. It should be highly seasoned since it will be served cold. Leave to cool, cover and chill for a few hours then serve sprinkled with chives or chervil.

Note

I have eaten *Vichyssoise* served with a spoonful of salted, whipped cream on top of each portion.

Nutritional Information		
One serving *Vichyssoise* with 3 slices of wholemeal bread		
Calories	519	Protein	11%
Fat	48%	Carbohydrate	41%
of which:		Vitamin A	>100%
monounsaturates	28%	Vitamin C	>100%
saturates	63%	Vitamin E	62%
polyunsaturates	9%		

SOUPE AU PISTOU

Rich Vegetable Soup flavoured with a Garlic, Basil and Cheese Paste

MIREILLE JOHNSTON

SERVES 4-6

The most exhilarating of soups, *Soupe au Pistou* is also the ultimate *potage de santé*, or health soup. It is generally served as the major part of a meal during the summer when there is an abundance of fresh vegetables; but in autumn or winter, leeks, dried haricot beans, pumpkin or turnips offer interesting alternatives and since the basil and cheese paste can be frozen (I always add the garlic at the last moment) *Soupe au Pistou* makes a fragrant and comforting starter at any time of the year.

In Nice, we like to prepare this soup with most of the vegetables diced into tiny cubes. In fact, in most marketplaces there are piles of freshly shelled white beans and neatly diced vegetables ready-prepared for the busy cook.

Soupe au Pistou can be prepared two or three days in advance. It can be served hot or at room temperature, and the basil mixture is always added to the warm broth at the table so that the heady potent scent of the herb can be enjoyed by all your guests. Remember that the quantity of basil and garlic depend on the quality and freshness of the ingredients and also on your personal taste, so keep tasting and correcting before stirring the pistou into the soup. It is always better to gather the basil leaves a few hours in advance so they lose some of their moisture.

FOR THE SOUP
225 g (8 oz) fresh, dried or semi-dried shelled white
or red and white haricot beans
4 onions
1 leek
1 tomato, skinned
4 potatoes
2 carrots
2 turnips
1 celery stick
4 courgettes
225 g (8 oz) green beans
3 tablespoons olive oil
2 bay leaves

a few fresh sage leaves
1.5 litres (3 pints) water
salt and freshly ground black pepper

FOR THE PISTOU
2 handfuls of fresh basil leaves
3 garlic cloves
4 tablespoons grated Gruyère or Parmesan
3 tablespoons olive oil

TO SERVE
grated Gruyère or Parmesan
crisp slices of bread

If you are using dried beans, soak them overnight in cold water. Drain and rinse. Place in a pan, cover with fresh water, bring to the boil and boil vigorously for 10 minutes then reduce the heat and simmer for about 1 hour until soft. Drain well.

Chop all the vegetables into 2.5 cm (1 in) pieces. Heat 2 tablespoons of the oil in a frying-pan and fry the onions and leek for 3 minutes. Add the tomato, potatoes, carrots, turnips and celery and cook for 10 minutes, stirring occasionally. Transfer to a large pan. Heat the remaining oil in the frying-pan and fry the courgettes, green beans, bay leaves and sage for a few minutes. Meanwhile, bring the water to the boil in a separate pan. Add the courgette mixture and the water to the vegetables with bay leaves and sage. Return to the boil and simmer, uncovered, for 30 minutes. Add the cooked haricot beans.

Meanwhile, prepare the pistou. Use a mortar and pestle to grind and pound the basil leaves, garlic, salt and pepper to a thick paste then add the cheese and oil. Alternatively, you can use a food processor. Pour the soup into a warm tureen and bring it to the table. Stir in the pistou then sprinkle a little cheese on top. Pass a bowl of grated cheese and a basket of crisp slices of bread around the table.

NUTRITIONAL INFORMATION			
One serving *Soupe au Pistou* with 2 slices of wholemeal bread and 1 tablespoon of Parmesan cheese to serve			
Calories	569	Protein	17%
Fat	30%	Carbohydrate	53%
of which:		Vitamin A	>100%
monounsaturates	51%	Vitamin C	>100%
saturates	30%	Vitamin E	38%
polyunsaturates	19%		

GAZPACHO

Chilled Tomato Soup

SOPHIE GRIGSON

SERVES 6

Gazpacho, the 'liquid salad', is a soup I never tire of. Pounding it by hand is a long tedious job, but with a processor preparing it is a matter of minutes. Remember that the proportions of vegetables and other ingredients that I give below are there merely to serve as a starting point. Tomatoes, peppers, garlic and all will vary in flavour from one batch to another, so it's important to keep tasting and to adjust the seasonings to compensate for any inadequacies. To intensify both the tomato flavour and colour of the soup you can replace some of the water with tomato juice, or add a tablespoon or two of tomato purée.

*750 g (1 ½lb) ripe, richly flavoured
tomatoes, skinned, deseeded and
roughly chopped
¾ cucumber, peeled and roughly chopped
1 large green pepper, deseeded and
roughly chopped
½ red onion, chopped
2-2½ tablespoons red wine vinegar
5 tablespoons olive oil
100 g (4 oz) fresh white breadcrumbs
2 cloves garlic, roughly chopped (optional)*

*½-1 teaspoon sugar
salt and pepper
300-450 ml (10-15 fl oz) iced water*

ANY OR ALL OF THE FOLLOWING TO SERVE
*diced, deseeded tomato
diced cucumber
diced red onion
diced red pepper
diced jamón serrano*

Put all ingredients in a processor with a small slurp of iced water. Process to a fairly smooth sludge (you may have to do this in 2 batches if your processor bowl is small). Gradually stir in enough water to give a soupy consistency, 300-450 ml (10-15 fl oz) should do it. Taste and adjust the seasoning, adding a little more salt, vinegar or sugar as necessary to highlight the flavours.

Chill, and adjust the seasoning again just before serving. Place all the garnishes in small bowls and pass around for people to help themselves.

NUTRITIONAL INFORMATION			
One serving *Gazpacho* with 2 slices of wholemeal bread			
Calories	283	Protein	12%
Fat	39%	Carbohydrate	49%
of which:		Vitamin A	28%
monounsaturates	66%	Vitamin C	100%
saturates	17%	Vitamin E	46%
polyunsaturates	17%		

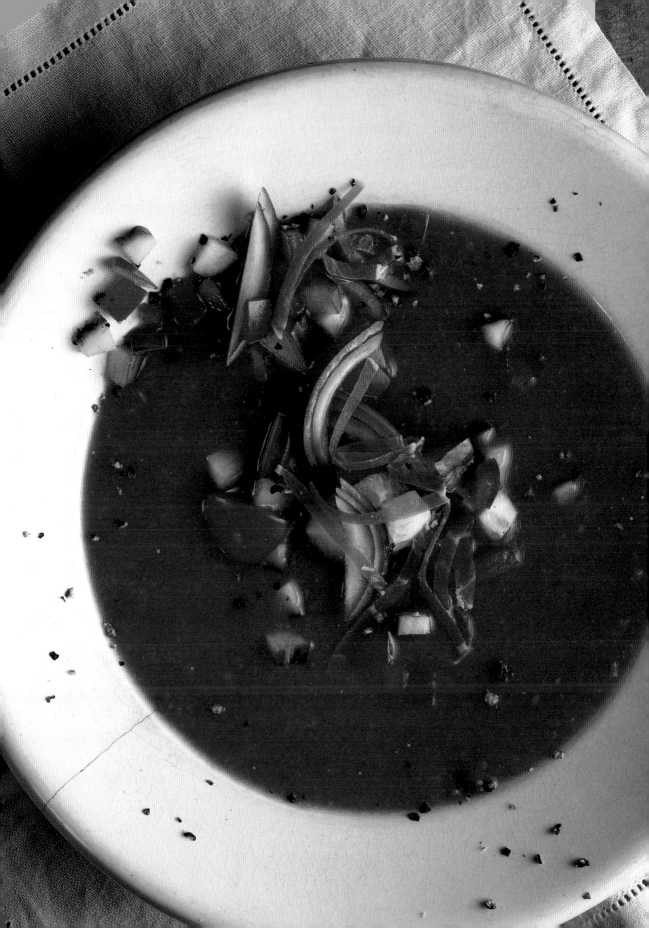

Starters

. . . .

CHAMPIGNONS FARCIS
Stuffed Mushrooms

CLAUDIA RODEN
SERVES 6

Those who are not keen on cooking snails but love the traditional garlic and parsley snail sauce will enjoy this Provençal dish.

500 g (1 lb) large flat mushrooms
olive oil
salt and pepper
65-75 g (2½-3 oz) parsley, finely chopped

2 slices of dry white bread, crusts removed
2 or more garlic cloves, crushed
2-3 tablespoons cognac (optional)

Wash the mushrooms briefly and cut off the stalks. Sauté in 2-3 tablespoons of oil for 5 minutes or until just tender, sprinkling with salt and pepper and turning them over once. Arrange, stem-side up, on a flat, heatproof dish.

To make the stuffing, chop the mushroom stalks and parsley and crumble the bread finely, or put them through a blender. Turn into a bowl and add as much garlic as you like and a little salt and pepper. Moisten with cognac, if using, and with 2-3 tablespoons olive oil and mix well. Press a little stuffing into each mushroom and grill for 5 minutes. Serve hot.

NUTRITIONAL INFORMATION			
One serving *Champignons Farcis* with 2 slices of wholemeal bread			
Calories	204	Protein	15%
Fat	31%	Carbohydrate	49%
of which:		Alcohol	5%
monounsaturates	62%	Vitamin A	15%
saturates	18%	Vitamin C	86%
polyunsaturates	20%	Vitamin E	12%

Lenticchie all'Olio

Lentils with Olive Oil

Valentina Harris

Serves 6

This very simple dish was actually served to us as a side dish in a small roadside trattoria in the Abruzzi. Lentils are used a great deal in the cooking of this region. The local lentils are tiny and dark brown, full of flavour. This dish is served throughout southern Italy and can also be prepared with other pulses.

300 g (11 oz) brown lentils, soaked overnight in cold water
½ teaspoon salt
6 tablespoons olive oil

½ red chilli pepper, deseeded and very finely chopped
2 cloves garlic, peeled and finely chopped
2 tablespoons chopped fresh parsley

Drain the lentils, wash carefully and cover with fresh water. Simmer, covered, for about 1-2 hours or until the lentils are completely soft. Mix the salt, oil, chilli, garlic and parsley together. Spoon the hot cooked lentils into 6 soup plates, then cover with the oil mixture and serve at once.

Note

If preferred, you can omit the chilli and/or the garlic and dress the lentils with just oil and chopped parsley.

NUTRITIONAL INFORMATION			
One serving *Lenticchie all'olio* with 2 slices of wholemeal bread			
Calories	406	Protein	17%
Fat	39%	Carbohydrate	44%
of which:		Vitamin A	2%
monounsaturates	68%	Vitamin C	16%
saturates	16%	Vitamin E	18%
polyunsaturates	16%		

PIEDMONT ROASTED PEPPERS

DELIA SMITH

SERVES 4 AS A STARTER

This recipe is quite simply stunning: hard to imagine how something so easily prepared can taste so good. Its history is colourful too. It was first discovered by Elizabeth David and published in her splendid book *Italian Food*. Then the Italian chef Franco Taruschio at the Walnut Tree Inn near Abergavenny cooked it there. Simon Hopkinson, who ate it at the Walnut Tree, put it on his menu at his great London restaurant Bibendum, where I ate it – which is how it comes to be here now for you to make and enjoy.

For this it is essential to use a good, solid, shallow roasting-tray 40 x 30 cm(16 x 12 inches): if the sides are too deep, the roasted vegetables won't get those lovely, nutty, toasted edges.

4 large red peppers (green are not suitable)
4 medium tomatoes
8 tinned anchovy fillets, drained
2 cloves garlic
8 dessertspoons Italian extra virgin olive oil
freshly milled black pepper

TO SERVE
I small bunch fresh basil leaves

Pre-heat the oven to gas mark 4, 180°C, 350°F.

Begin by cutting the peppers in half and removing the seeds but leaving the stalks intact (they're not edible but they do look attractive and they help the pepper halves to keep their shape). Lay the pepper halves in a lightly oiled roasting-tray. Now put the tomatoes in a bowl and pour boiling water over them. Leave them for 1 minute, then drain them and slip the skins off, using a cloth to protect your hands. Then cut the tomatoes in quarters and place two quarters in each pepper half.

After that snip one anchovy fillet per pepper half into rough pieces and add to the tomatoes. Peel the garlic cloves, slice them thinly and divide the slices equally among the tomatoes and anchovies. Now spoon 1 dessertspoon of olive oil into each pepper, season with freshly milled pepper (but no salt because of the anchovies) and place the tray on a

high shelf in the oven for the peppers to roast for 50 minutes-1 hour.

Then transfer the cooked peppers to a serving-dish, with all the precious juices poured over, and garnish with a few scattered basil leaves. These do need good bread to go with them as the juices are sublime. Focaccia with olive would be perfect.

NUTRITIONAL INFORMATION			
One serving *Piedmont Roasted Peppers* with 2 slices of wholemeal bread			
Calories	321	Protein	10%
Fat	52%	Carbohydrate	38%
of which:		Vitamin A	>100%
monounsaturates	69%	Vitamin C	>100%
saturates	16%	Vitamin E	46%
polyunsaturates	15%		

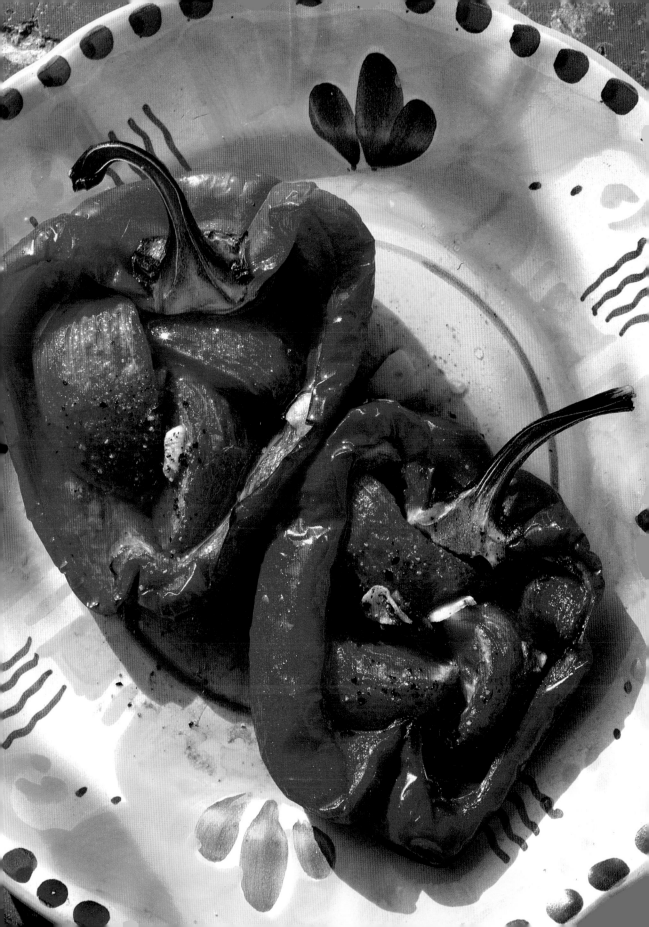

HARENGS SAURS
Marinated Cured Herring Fillets

MIREILLE JOHNSTON
SERVES 4

A true bistro staple that is a particular speciality of Boulogne. Just a look at the big brown or white dishes of *Harengs Saurs* on the table will tell you whether you are in a serious place or not.

This is one of the easiest dishes to prepare at home, and it will keep covered in the fridge for at least one week. *Harengs Saurs* are salted and smoked whole; for convenience and availability, kipper fillets can be substituted for them.

8 harengs saurs or kipper fillets,
each about 13 cm (5 in) long
1 onion, sliced
1 carrot, sliced
2 bay leaves
1 sprig of fresh thyme
1 lemon, sliced
10 black peppercorns

about 300 ml (8-10 fl oz) mixed olive oil and
groundnut oil
fresh flatleaf parsley leaves

TO SERVE
Good country bread or warm sliced potatoes seasoned
with oil, vinegar, parsley or chives and salt.

Place the kipper fillets in the bottom of an attractive, round or rectangular, white china or brown earthenware dish. Cover with the onion, carrot, bay leaves, thyme, lemon and peppercorns. Pour over sufficient oil to cover generously. Cover the dish with foil or cling film and leave in the fridge for at least 2 days, turning the fillets over twice during that time. Sprinkle over the parsley and serve at room temperature with the bread or potatoes.

Variation
Add 1 or 2 crushed garlic cloves an hour before serving.

NUTRITIONAL INFORMATION			
One serving *Harengs Saurs* served with a quarter of a baguette			
Calories	846	Protein	15%
Fat	58%	Carbohydrate	27%
of which:		Vitamin A	58%
monounsaturates	63%	Vitamin C	46%
saturates	22%	Vitamin E	>40%
polyunsaturates	15%		

PÂTÉ DI OLIVE NERE

Black Olive Pâté

VALENTINA HARRIS

SERVES 8

This intensely flavoured olive spread first became popular in the southern immigrant areas of Piedmont, and it was the incomers who first introduced the idea to the rather strait-laced natives of Turin. It has since become a firm favourite in even the most aristocratic families! It makes a delicious snack to savour before a meal and is traditionally served with ice-cold, fairly acidic white wine to offset the slightly cloying flavour of the olives. It is important to use juicy olives with plenty of flavour in this recipe – not the bitter calamata olives. In the summer months, many people add aubergine pulp to the mixture (see Variation below).

225 g (8 oz) black olives
grated rind and juice of ½ lemon, strained
1 large tablespoon best-quality olive oil
50 g (2 oz) softened butter
(preferably unsalted)
20 g (¾ oz) very fresh white breadcrumbs

pinch of salt
generous grinding of black pepper

To SERVE
Thin slices of bread, lightly toasted then coated with just a sheen of olive oil, applied with a brush.

If the olives are not stoned, remove the stones with an olive pitter or very sharp knife. Chop them as finely as possible using a *mezzaluna* or a sharp knife, then put them through a mincer two or three times using the finest blade.

Alternatively, whizz them in a food processor for about 30 seconds at high speed. When you have a smooth purée, stir in the lemon juice and the olive oil, then the butter and breadcrumbs, and finally the grated lemon rind, salt and pepper. Do be generous with the pepper! Stir and stir until you have a very light, almost fluffy texture with no lumps. Taste and adjust the seasoning – you may like to add more lemon juice. Spoon into small individual bowls and refrigerate for a minimum of 3 hours before serving.

Serve with thin slices of toast.

Variation

Instead of 225 g (8 oz) olives, use 100 g (4 oz) olives and 100 g (4 oz) aubergines. Purée the olives as above. Slice the aubergines and grill them until dry and papery. Push them through a sieve or blend in the food processor to a smooth purée. Mix with the olive purée and proceed as above.

NUTRITIONAL INFORMATION			
One serving *Pâté di Olive Nere* with 2 slices of wholemeal toast coated with olive oil			
Calories	259	Protein	11%
Fat	47%	Carbohydrate	42%
of which:		Vitamin A	13%
monunsaturates	49%	Vitamin C	36%
saturates	39%	Vitamin E	20%
polyunsaturates	12%		

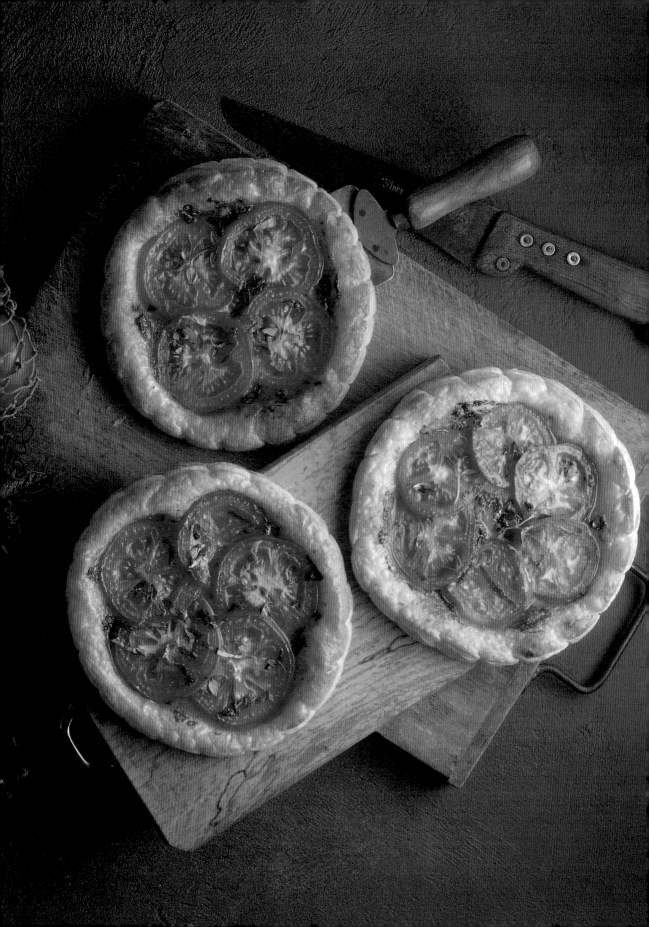

Tarte Fine à la Tomate et au Pistou

Puff Pastry Tart with Tomatoes and Pistou

Sophie Grigson

SERVES 6

A *tarte fine* is a thin disc of puff pastry, covered with a savoury or sweet filling and baked quickly in a hot oven. This recipe, from French chef, Michel Guérard, pairs the thin crisp pastry with tomatoes, basil and olive oil. With richly flavoured tomatoes, it is the most heavenly first course. The only drawback is that you will probably have to cook the *tartes fines* in relays, unless you have an extremely large oven.

2 tablespoons finely chopped fresh basil
120 ml (4 fl oz) extra virgin olive oil
2 tablespoons tomato purée
450 g (1 lb) puff pastry
6 ripe, medium-sized tomatoes

salt and freshly ground white pepper
sugar
½ teaspoon fresh thyme leaves
12 extra basil leaves, roughly torn up

Mix the chopped basil with 1½ tablespoons of the olive oil and set aside for 5-10 minutes, then mix with the tomato purée. Roll out the puff pastry very thinly (it's probably easiest to do this in 2 halves) and cut out six 20-cm (8-inch) diameter circles. Prick all over with a fork and lay them on oiled baking sheets. Spread the basil and tomato purée mixture over the circles, using a brush, leaving a 1-cm (½-inch) border all the way round the edges.

Pre-heat the oven to gas mark 8, 230°C, 450°F. Slice the tomatoes as thinly as you can. Discard the seeds and juice. Arrange the tomato rings on the pastry. Season with salt, pepper and a little sugar. Scatter over the thyme. Bake in the oven. After 5 minutes, brush the tarts generously with olive oil and return to the oven for a final 5-8 minutes until nicely browned. Serve immediately, scattered with a few torn up basil leaves.

NUTRITIONAL INFORMATION			
One serving *Tarte Fine à la Tomate et au Pistou* with 2 slices of wholemeal bread			
Calories	715	Protein	5%
Fat	65%	Carbohydrate	30%
of which:		Vitamin A	46%
monounsaturates	54%	Vitamin C	38%
saturates	33%	Vitamin E	100%
polyunsaturates	13%		

CROSTINI DI POLLO E FEGATO

Chicken and Calf's Liver Crostini

VALENTINA HARRIS

SERVES 4

This recipe is one of my own and comes from Tuscany. Many variations are to be found in different parts of the region but I always come back to this one. Crostini are simply pieces of bread covered with a delicious savoury topping – ideal with a pre-dinner glass of wine.

½ onion, chopped
1 carrot, chopped
1 stick celery, chopped
1 tablespoon finely chopped parsley
3 tablespoons olive oil
40 g (1½ oz) unsalted butter
1 chicken liver, trimmed and washed
100 g (4 oz) calf's liver, trimmed and washed

2 tablespoons dry white wine
1 heaped tablespoon tomato purée diluted with about 4 tablespoons hot water
salt and pepper
25 g (1 oz) capers, rinsed and finely chopped
4 or 8 thin slices crusty white or brown bread

Fry the onion, carrot, celery and parsley in the olive oil and half the butter. Cook until the onion is soft, then add the chicken and calf's livers. Stir and add the wine. Allow to evaporate for 2-3 minutes, then add the diluted tomato purée. Season with a little salt and pepper, add 2-3 tablespoons water, cover and simmer for about 20 minutes.

Remove from the heat, lift the livers out of the sauce and mince or process them until smooth. Return the liver purée to the pan and stir in the rest of the butter and the capers. Heat through and remove from the heat, but keep warm.

Spread the bread generously with the liver mixture and serve at once.

NUTRITIONAL INFORMATION			
One serving *Crostini di Pollo e Fegato* with 2 slices of wholemeal bread			
Calories	362	Protein	13%
Fat	57%	Carbohydrate	29%
of which:		Alcohol	1%
monounsaturates	50%	Vitamin A	>100%
saturates	12%	Vitamin C	58%
polyunsaturates	38%	Vitamin E	28%

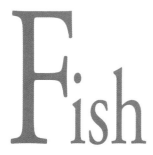

Fish

Salmone al Pesto

Salmon with Pesto

Valentina Harris

SERVES 6

As an alternative to cooking salmon in this way, you could cover the fish in pesto and wrap it in foil. Place the foil parcels under the grill or in a hot oven at gas mark 6, 200°C, 400°F, and cook them for about 5 or 6 minutes before serving them for your guests to unwrap at the table.

*12 very small salmon tail fillets or
salmon steaks
1 jar very good quality pesto sauce
1 wine glass dry white wine*

*3 tablespoons olive oil
salt
freshly ground black pepper
4 leaves fresh basil*

Arrange the fish in a shallow bowl. Whisk the pesto with the wine and oil until the sauce has emulsified completely. Pour the mixture over the fish and season to taste with salt and pepper. Leave to marinate in a cool place, but not the fridge, for about 5 hours, turning the fish occasionally.

Heat a skillet or heavy non-stick pan rubbed lightly with olive oil. Cook the fish briefly for about 4 minutes each side, turning frequently. While the fish is cooking, spoon over the pesto sauce so that by the time the fish is cooked, all the sauce is in the pan. Arrange the fish and sauce on a warmed serving platter, and serve garnished with basil leaves.

NUTRITIONAL INFORMATION			
One serving *Salmone al Pesto* with 4 new potatoes, broccoli and 1 slice of wholemeal bread			
Calories	566	Protein	20%
Fat	49%	Carbohydrate	31%
of which:		Vitamin A	44%
monounsaturates	27%	Vitamin C	46%
saturates	23%	Vitamin E	>100%
polyunsaturates	50%		

Recommended Red Wines: Bourgueil, Chinon, Kekfrancos, chilled Pinotage and young Tempranillo
White Wine: Alsatian Tokay Pinot Gris.

Brandade

Salt Cod and Potato Purée

Mireille Johnston

SERVES 6

Dried salt cod has been a staple of French Mediterranean cookery for centuries. It was taken to Provence and Languedoc by Norwegian and other traders from northern waters. The process which transforms a hard, dry, grey piece of fish into *Brandade*, an ivory, fluffy mousse, is not a complicated one. Traditional *Brandade* required a great amount of olive oil, but the recipe I use here contains less oil but more milk and potatoes, so is lighter and less rich. When it is served as a white pyramid, sprinkled with black olives and surrounded by crisp croûtons it makes a splendid, fragrant dish. *Brandade* can be prepared in advance. Warm through gently and beat in 2 tablespoons of warm milk or cream.

750 g (1½ lb) dried salt cod
2 bay leaves
1 onion, studded with 1 clove
450 g (1 lb) potatoes, unpeeled
300 ml (10 fl oz) milk
250 ml (8 fl oz) olive oil
3 garlic cloves, crushed
2 teaspoons freshly grated nutmeg

juice of 1 lemon or 1 orange
freshly ground white pepper
2 tablespoons Niçoise or black Greek olives, halved if large, stoned
3 slices good, firm bread prepared as triangular croûtons
1 tablespoon chopped fresh parsley

Place the dried salt cod in a large pan or basin and cover with cold water. Soak for at least 24 hours, changing the water 5 or 6 times.

Drain the dried salt cod then place on an upturned heatproof plate or small dish in an enamelled or stainless steel saucepan and cover with cold water. Add the bay leaves and onion and bring slowly to the boil. Lower the heat, poach for 3 minutes, then turn off the heat and leave the cod to cool in the water. Drain well, remove the skin and any bones and flake the flesh with a fork.

Cook the potatoes in boiling water until soft. Drain well, leave to cool then peel and press through a sieve.

Warm the milk and all except 1½ tablespoons of the oil in separate pans. Place a few pieces of cod in a food processor and mix briefly. Add the garlic and more flaked cod, and continue processing, alternately pouring in milk and oil, and adding cod until you have a smooth ivory purée. Transfer to a bowl and gradually beat in the potato. Add nutmeg, lemon or orange juice and pepper.

Transfer to a warm shallow dish. Sprinkle over the remaining olive oil, stir and mound into a dome. Arrange the olives in the centre of the dome. Dip the tips of the triangular croûtons into the *Brandade*, then into chopped parsley and place round the dish.

NUTRITIONAL INFORMATION			
One serving *Brandade* with courgettes, carrots and 1 slice of wholemeal bread			
Calories	863	Protein	25%
Fat	49%	Carbohydrate	26%
of which:		Vitamin A	>100%
monounsaturates	68%	Vitamin C	>100%
saturates	18%	Vitamin E	60%
polyunsaturates	14%		

Recommended Red Wines: Moroccan red, young reds from the Alentejo and Ribatejo, Pinotage, chilled young Tempranillo.
White Wines: Australian semillon, South African sauvignon blanc, New Zealand chardonnay.

DAURADE AU FOUR

Baked Bream with Fennel, Lemon and Herbs

MIREILLE JOHNSTON

SERVES 4

An uncomplicated dish, but the ingredients must be fresh.

4 tablespoons olive oil
3 onions, thinly sliced
1 fennel bulb, trimmed, thinly sliced
into rounds
about 10 sprigs of fresh parsley
2 bay leaves
salt and freshly ground black pepper
1.25 kg (2 ¾ lb) bream, halibut or bass,
filleted

4 tomatoes, seeded and sliced
4 teaspoons fennel seeds or aniseeds
1 lemon, sliced
5 tablespoons dry white wine
3 or 4 large iceberg coarse lettuce leaves
juice of 1 lemon

Pre-heat the oven to gas mark 4, 180°C, 350°F.

Heat 2 tablespoons of olive oil in a frying-pan, add the onions and fennel and cook over a moderate heat, stirring occasionally, for about 5 minutes until beginning to soften.

Place half of the onions and fennel, the parsley and 1 bay leaf in a baking dish. Sprinkle with a little salt and pepper. Lay half of the fish on top, skin-side down, sprinkle with salt, pepper and olive oil. Place the remaining fish on top, skin-side up. Cover with the tomatoes, remaining onions, fennel and bay leaf, the fennel seeds or aniseeds and the lemon slices. Pour over the wine and a little olive oil.

Lay a few lettuce leaves loosely on top and bake in the oven for about 25 minutes until the flesh is milky when tested with the tip of a knife. Discard the lettuce leaves. Using 2 fish slices, carefully transfer the fish to a warm serving dish. Sprinkle with

the lemon juice and a little pepper, then trickle over the remaining olive oil and serve immediately.

NUTRITIONAL INFORMATION			
One serving *Daurade au Four* with a green salad and 1 teaspoon vinaigrette			
Calories	578	Protein	5%
Fat	30%	Carbohydrate	63%
of which:		Alcohol	2%
monounsaturates	72%	Vitamin A	20%
saturates	15%	Vitamin C	>100%
polyunsaturates	13%	Vitamin E	42%

Recommended Red Wines: Chilled Kekfrancos or Hungarian country reds.
White Wines: Vin de Pays d'Oc chardonnay, South African chardonnays.

SARDINES EN BROCHETTES

Sardine and Pepper Brochettes

MIREILLE JOHNSTON

SERVES 1

I discovered this simple dish on the charming island of Noirmoutier, in the Atlantic ocean just off the Vendée coast. Noirmoutier is a holiday resort which resembles a Greek island, with its stark windmills and whitewashed, blue-shuttered cottages. The sardines were prepared using the local fragrant sea salt, newly harvested and smelling faintly of violets. They were served with the renowned Noirmountier Charlotte potatoes.

From Brittany to Provence there are endless ways of using sardines – raw with lemon and oil, marinated in lemon juice, grilled, stuffed and fried. In this dish they are treated very simply. Dipping them in sea salt adds flavour and makes them easier to fold onto the skewers.

4 sardines, each weighing about
100 g (4 oz)
about 75 g (3 oz) coarse sea salt
½ teaspoon dried thyme
freshly ground white pepper

½ red pepper, cut into 4 cm (1½ in) pieces
½ green pepper, cut into 4 cm (1½in) pieces
¼ onion, separated into layers, cut into 4 cm
(1½ in) pieces
1½ tablespoon olive oil

Pre-heat the grill. Working from tail to head and using a knife, scrape the scales from the sardines. Slit along the underside of each fish then remove the intestines. Cut off the heads. Open out each fish and place, skin-side up, on a board. With a thumb, press lightly along the centre of the back of one fish, then turn the fish over and lift away the backbone. Leave the boned fish in coarse sea salt for 30 seconds. Remove from the salt and carefully brush off all the excess. Sprinkle over a little thyme and pepper.

Brush the peppers and onion with olive oil and sprinkle with sea salt and pepper. Skewer sardines, red pepper and green pepper and onion alternately along a skewer until all the ingredients have been used. Grill for 5-8 minutes, turning a few times.

NUTRITIONAL INFORMATION			
One serving *Sardines en Brochettes* with 4 new potatoes, and a third of a baguette			
Calories	698	Protein	10%
Fat	26%	Carbohydrate	64%
of which:		Vitamin A	>100%
monounsaturates	63%	Vitamin C	>100%
saturates	19%	Vitamin E	44%
polyunsaturates	18%		

Recommended Red Wines: Chilled Romanian Pinot Noir, Fitou, Mas de Daumas Gassac blanc.
White Wines: Chilean sauvignon blanc, New Zealand sauvignon blanc.

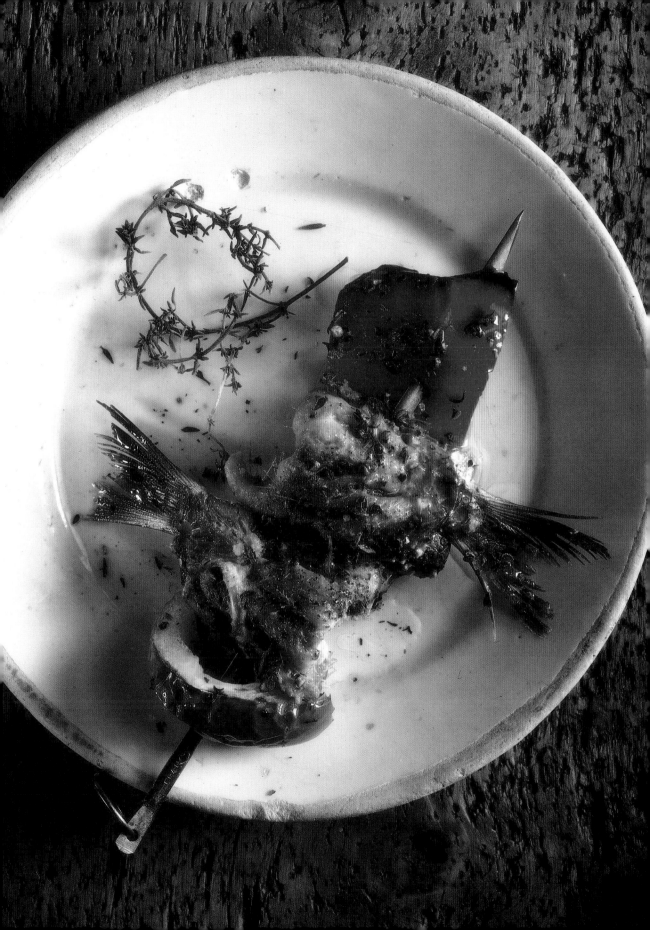

GAMBAS AL AJILLO

Garlic Prawns

CLAUDIA RODEN

SERVES 4

This popular Spanish *tapa* is traditionally cooked in a small earthenware dish over the fire but it works perfectly in a frying-pan. It cooks in an instant and is absolutely delicious.

3 garlic cloves, finely chopped
1 small dried or fresh chilli pepper, deseeded and
chopped, or a pinch of cayenne
4 tablespoons olive oil

250 g (8 oz) shelled prawns
salt
small bunch of parsley, finely chopped
lemon wedges

Fry the garlic and pepper in the oil. Add the prawns as soon as the garlic begins to colour. Season with salt and continue to fry over a high heat for 1-2 minutes. Serve sizzling hot, preferably straight from the pan, sprinkled with parsley and accompanied by lemon wedges.

Recommended Red Wine: chilled Barbaresco.
White Wines: Chilled fino sherry, Côtes du Rhône.

NUTRITIONAL INFORMATION			
One serving *Gambas al Ajillo* with a third of a baguette			
Calories	526	Protein	14%
Fat	33%	Carbohydrate	53%
of which:		Vitamin A	3%
monounsaturates	66%	Vitamin C	36%
saturates	18%	Vitamin E	16%
polyunsaturates	16%		

CHILLED MARINATED TROUT WITH FENNEL

DELIA SMITH

SERVES 2

This makes a very appropriate main course for a warm day. It's a doddle to prepare and it has the advantage of being cooked and left to marinate, so that when the time comes you have literally nothing to do but serve it. We like this either with a plain mixed-leaf salad or with a pesto rice salad.

2 x 225 g (8 oz) bright fresh rainbow trout
450 g (1 lb) ripe red tomatoes, skinned
and chopped
1 bulb fennel, trimmed and sliced
(green tops reserved)

225 ml (8 fl oz) dry white wine
1 clove garlic, finely chopped
1 small onion, finely chopped
¾ teaspoon whole black peppercorns
¾ teaspoon coriander seeds

½ teaspoon fennel seeds
2 tablespoons extra virgin olive oil
1 tablespoon white wine vinegar
1 tablespoon lemon juice
½ teaspoon fresh oregano
salt and freshly milled black pepper

For the Garnish
2 small spring onions, finely chopped
2 tablespoons chopped parsley
grated zest of 1 lemon
fennel tops

You will also need a 25 cm (10-inch) frying-pan or wide, shallow pan.

Begin by washing the fish and drying it with kitchen paper. Then warm the frying-pan over a gentle heat, crush the peppercorns, coriander and fennel seeds in a mortar, add the crushed spices and let them dry-roast for about 1 minute to draw out the flavours. Then add the olive oil, garlic and onion and let them cook gently for about 5 minutes or until the onion is pale gold.

Next add the tomatoes, lemon juice, wine vinegar and white wine, stir and, when it begins to bubble, season with salt and pepper and add the oregano. Now add the sliced fennel to the pan, followed by the trout, basting the fish with the juices. Put a timer on and give the whole thing 10 minutes' gentle simmering. After that use a fish slice and fork to turn each fish over carefully on to its other side – don't prod it or anything like that or the flesh will break. Then give it another 10 minutes' cooking on the other side.

After that gently remove the trout to a shallow serving-dish, spoon the sauce all over, cool, cover with clingfilm and leave them in a cool place. If you want to make this dish the day before, that's OK provided you keep it refrigerated and remove it an hour before serving. Either way sprinkle each trout with the garnish (made by simply combining all the ingredients together) before taking to the table.

Note
If the weather's chilly, this dish is excellent served warm with tiny new potatoes and a leafy salad.

NUTRITIONAL INFORMATION			
One serving *Chilled Marinated Trout with Fennel* with 4 new potatoes and a green salad with 1 teaspoon of vinaigrette			
Calories	786	Protein	31%
Fat	36%	Carbohydrate	24%
of which:		Alcohol	9%
monounsaturates	59%	Vitamin A	84%
saturates	18%	Vitamin C	>100%
polyunsaturates	23%	Vitamin E	86%

Recommended Red Wines: chilled Chinon and Bourgueil.
White Wines: Côtes du Rhône and Châteauneuf-du-Pape.

Mussels with Lemon Dressing

Claudia Roden

SERVES 4-6

The simplest way of dealing with mussels is also one of the most attractive.

2 kg (4 lb) mussels
300 ml (10 fl oz) olive oil
juice of 2-3 lemons

salt and pepper
2 garlic cloves, crushed (optional)
large bunch of parsley, finely chopped

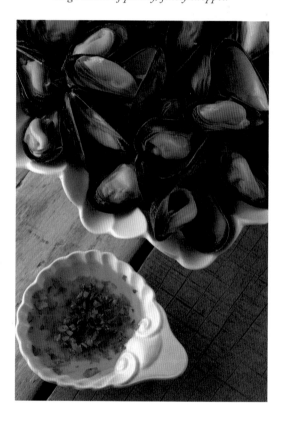

Clean the mussels and steam them open. Let them cool or serve them at once.

To make the sauce, beat the oil and lemon juice with the rest of the ingredients. It is usual to pour some over each serving but I think it is easier and less wasteful to provide little bowls of sauce on each plate for people to dip their mussels in.

NUTRITIONAL INFORMATION			
One serving *Mussels with Lemon Dressing* with 3 slices of wholemeal bread			
Calories	900	Protein	27%
Fat	58%	Carbohydrate	15%
of which:		Vitamin A	2%
monounsaturates	68%	Vitamin C	81%
saturates	17%	Vitamin E	54%
polyunsaturates	15%		

Recommended Red Wine: chilled Tempranillo.
White Wine: Vin de Pays des Côtes de Gascogne.

Poultry

POLLO ALLA SALVIA

Pan-roasted Chicken with Sage

VALENTINA HARRIS

SERVES 6

A marvellously simple chicken dish, this tastes absolutely wonderful. It is very good served with carrots and mashed potatoes.

1 heaped tablespoon unsalted butter
2 tablespoons olive oil
6 large chicken joints, trimmed
1 large wine glass dry white wine

50 g (2 oz) prosciutto crudo, cut into slivers
1 sprig of fresh sage, roughly chopped
salt
freshly ground black pepper

Heat the butter and oil in a large frying pan and fry the chicken joints gently until dark golden all over. Drain off as much of the fat as possible, pour over the wine and boil off the alcohol for about 2 minutes. Sprinkle on the prosciutto and sage and season generously with salt and pepper. Mix everything together thoroughly, cover and simmer gently for about 45 minutes, basting occasionally with a little water if the chicken appears to be drying out too much. Serve at once.

NUTRITIONAL INFORMATION			
One serving *Pollo alla Salvia* with mashed potato and carrots			
Calories	419	Protein	23%
Fat	40%	Carbohydrate	34%
of which:		Alcohol	3%
monounsaturates	39%	Vitamin A	>100%
saturates	50%	Vitamin C	52%
polyunsaturates	11%	Vitamin E	26%

Recommended Red Wines: Barolo, Aglianico del Vulture, Ribera del Duero.

Coq au Vin

Delia Smith

SERVES 6-8

A truly authentic coq au vin is made, obviously, with a cock bird, and some of the blood goes into the sauce which, by the time it reaches the table, is a rich, almost black colour. In Britain we make a less authentic adaptation, but it makes a splendid dinner party dish.

1 x 2.25 kg (5 lb) chicken, cut into 8 joints
25 g (1 oz) butter
1 tablespoon oil
22r g (8 oz) unsmoked streaky bacon in one piece
16 button onions
2 cloves garlic, crushed
2 sprigs of fresh thyme
2 bay leaves

725 ml (1¼) pints red wine
225 g (8 oz) dark-gilled mushrooms
a butter and flour paste made with 1 rounded table-spoon softened butter and 1 tablespoon plain flour
salt and freshly milled black pepper

A large flameproof pot, wide and shallow to take the joints in one layer.

Melt the butter with the oil in a frying pan, and fry the chicken joints, skin side down, until they are nicely golden; then turn them and colour the other side. You may have to do this in three or four batches – don't overcrowd the pan. Remove the joints from the pan with a draining-spoon, and place them in a large cooking pot. The pot should be large enough for the joints to be arranged in one layer yet deep enough so that they can be completely covered with liquid later. The pot must also be flameproof.

Now de-rind and cut the bacon into fairly small cubes, brown them also in the frying pan and add them to the chicken, then finally brown the onions a little and add them too. Next place the crushed cloves of garlic and the sprigs of thyme among the chicken pieces, season with freshly milled pepper and just a little salt, and pop in a couple of bay leaves.

Pour in the wine, put a lid on the pot and simmer gently for 45-60 minutes or until the chicken is tender. During the last 15 minutes of the cooking, add the mushrooms and stir them into the liquid.

Remove the chicken, bacon, onions and mushrooms and place them on a warmed serving dish. Keep warm. (Discard the bay leaves and thyme at this stage.)

Now bring the liquid to a fast boil and reduce it by about one-third. Next, add the butter and flour paste

to the liquid. Bring it to the boil, whisking all the time until the sauce has thickened, then serve the chicken with the sauce poured over. If you like, sprinkle some chopped parsley over the chicken and make it look pretty.

Note

The results are different but every bit as delicious if you use cider instead of wine, but it must be dry cider. I also like now to give this half its cooking time the day before, let it cool, then refrigerate and give it the other half of the cooking time before serving. At the half-cooked stage, turn the chicken pieces over so that they can absorb all the lovely flavours overnight.

NUTRITIONAL INFORMATION			
One serving *Coq au Vin* with rice			
Calories	806	Protein	26%
Fat	34%	Carbohydrate	31%
of which:		Alcohol	9%
monounsaturates	44%	Vitamin A	11%
saturates	50%	Vitamin C	36%
polyunsaturates	6%	Vitamin E	22%

Drink the red wine used to cook the bird: Oregon Merlot, Mexican cabernet sauvignon, Pinotage, Madiran, Bandol, Cahors.

Chicken with Sherry Vinegar and Tarragon Sauce

Delia Smith

Serves 4

This is my adaptation of a classic French dish called *poulet au vinaigre*. It's very simple to make: the chicken is flavoured with tarragon leaves and simmered in a mixture of sherry vinegar and medium sherry without a lid, so that the liquid cooks down to a glossy, concentrated sauce. Serve some well-chilled Fino sherry as an aperitif – perfect for a warm summer's evening.

1.75 kg (1 x 3½ lb) chicken, jointed into 8 pieces, or
you could use 4 bone-in chicken breast portions
150 ml (5 fl oz) sherry vinegar
425 ml (15 fl oz) medium-dry Amontillado sherry
12 shallots, peeled and left whole
4 cloves garlic, peeled and left whole
2 tablespoons olive oil
2 tablespoons fresh tarragon leaves

1 heaped tablespoon crème fraîche
salt and freshly milled black pepper

To Garnish
8 small sprigs of fresh tarragon

You will also need a large, roomy frying-pan 23 cm (9 inches) in diameter.

First of all heat the oil in the frying-pan and season the chicken joints with salt and pepper. Then, when the oil begins to shimmer, fry the chicken (in two batches) to brown well: remove the first batch to a plate while you tackle the second. Each joint needs to be a lovely golden-brown colour. When the second batch is ready, remove it to the plate to join the rest. Then add the shallots to the pan, brown these a little, and finally add the garlic cloves to colour slightly.

Now turn the heat down, return the chicken pieces to the pan, scatter the tarragon leaves all over, then pour in the vinegar and sherry. Let it all simmer for a bit, then turn the heat to a very low setting so that the whole thing barely bubbles for 45 minutes. Half-way through turn the chicken pieces over to allow the other sides to sit in the sauce.

When they're ready, remove them to a warm serving-dish (right side up) along with the shallots and garlic. The sauce will by now have reduced and concentrated, so all you do is whisk the crème fraîche into it, taste and season as required, then pour the sauce all over the chicken and scatter with the sprigs of tarragon. This is lovely served with tiny new potatoes tossed in herbs and some fresh shelled peas.

Nutritional Information			
One serving *Chicken with Sherry Vinegar and Tarragon Sauce* with 4 new potatoes and peas			
Calories	767	Protein	34%
Fat	27%	Carbohydrate	25%
of which:		Alcohol	14%
monounsaturates	51%	Vitamin A	–
saturates	30%	Vitamin C	46%
polyunsaturates	19%	Vitamin E	18%

Recommended Red Wines: Château Musar, Californian Zinfandel, Australian shiraz, Bandol.

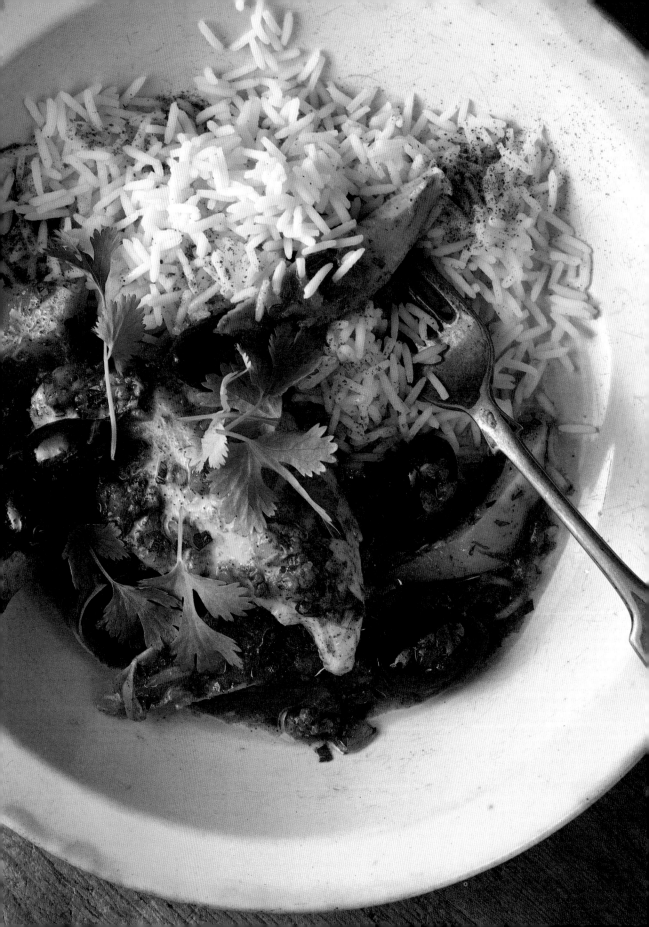

Djaj Mqualli

Chicken with Preserved Lemons and Olives

Claudia Roden

SERVES 4

The cooking of all the North African countries derives from Morocco because the empires which spread throughout the area were centred there. Moroccan chicken with preserved lemon and olives is one of the most popular dishes. Lemons which are preserved in salt lose their sharpness and become soft and mellow. Their flavour is complemented in this recipe by that of olives, soaked in water and then blanched to remove any saltiness or bitterness. As in many Moroccan chicken dishes, the mashed livers are used to give body to the sauce.

1 chicken, including the liver, weighing about
1.5 kg (3 lb)
½ teaspoon ginger
1½ teaspoons cinnamon
large pinch of saffron-coloured powder
salt
white pepper
3 tablespoons sunflower oil

2-3 garlic cloves
1 large onion, finely chopped
large bunch of parsley, finely chopped
large bunch of coriander, finely chopped
peel of 1 preserved lemon or 2 preserved limes, rinsed
and cut into small pieces
50 g (2 oz) pinky-green or brown olives, soaked in
2 changes of water for 1 hour

Clean the chicken. Put the ginger, cinnamon, saffron, a pinch of salt and pepper in a large pan with about 700 ml (1¼ pints) of water and the oil. Stir well, then add the chicken with its liver and the remaining ingredients, except the preserved lemon or lime peel and the olives. Cook, covered, for 45 minutes, turning it over occasionally and adding more water if necessary. Add the peel and the drained and rinsed olives. Cook for a further 15 minutes or until the chicken is so tender that the flesh easily comes away from the bone. Remove the liver, mash it, then return it to the pan to thicken the sauce, which should be greatly reduced but not too dry.

Transfer the chicken to a serving plate and pour the sauce over the top. Serve hot.

NUTRITIONAL INFORMATION			
One serving *Djaj Mqualli* with rice and 1 slice of wholemeal bread			
Calories	557	Protein	38%
Fat	39%	Carbohydrate	23%
of which:		Vitamin A	>100%
monounsaturates	33%	Vitamin C	>100%
saturates	23%	Vitamin E	72%
polyunsaturates	44%		

Recommended Red Wines: Château Musar, Cahors

Djaj Meshwi

Grilled Spring Chicken

Claudia Roden

SERVES 2

Restaurants along the Nile such as the Casino des Pigeons are famed for grilled young pigeons and quail which are great delicacies in Egypt. Baby chicken is the standby when pigeons and quail are out of season. Pigeons in Britain are different birds altogether and not suitable for grilling. Quail are excellent and you should use them when you can, but this recipe is for spring chicken (poussin), which is readily available and which is at its best when cooked this way. If you cannot cook on a charcoal or wood fire do them under the grill.

2 poussins
4 tablespoons olive oil
juice of 1 lemon
1-4 garlic cloves, crushed

pepper
2 tablespoons butter (optional)
salt
bunch of parsley, finely chopped

Lay the poussins breast down and split them open all along the backbone. Crack the breastbone and open the birds out. Cut the wing and leg joints just enough to spread them out. Turn the poussins over and pound each one flat so they cook evenly.

Mix the oil and lemon juice with the garlic and pepper in a bowl. Marinate the poussins in a cool place for an hour or two, turning them over once.

Place the birds on an oiled grill 7.5 cm (3 in) from the heat, skin-side down, and cook for 8-10 minutes until the skin has turned brown. Brush with the marinade or with melted butter, sprinkle the poussins with salt and turn them over. Cook for about 15 minutes and turn again, if necessary, until the juice from a thigh when you prick it with a fork is no longer pink. Serve sprinkled with parsley.

Note about quails

Split quails down the back, marinate and cook as above but only for 5-6 minutes. You can also wrap the quails in vine leaves – fresh ones or preserved in brine – as a protection against drying out. The leaves give them a distinctive flavour. (Leaves in brine should be soaked in water first.)

Marinade variations

• Syrians like to add 1 tablespoon thyme.
• Omit the lemon juice, but add 2 teaspoons paprika, 1 teaspoon cumin and a pinch of cayenne, and serve sprinkled with chopped coriander for a Moroccan flavour.
• One of my favourites is also Egyptian: put 1 onion in a blender with 1 teaspoon cumin, ½ teaspoon coriander, ½ teaspoon cinnamon, a pinch each of allspice, ginger and nutmeg, and salt and pepper. Blend to a paste and spread this on the meat.

NUTRITIONAL INFORMATION			
One serving *Djaj Meshwi* with a third of a baguette and a green salad with 1 teaspoon of vinaigrette			
Calories	905	Protein	29%
Fat	40%	Carbohydrate	31%
of which:		Vitamin A	11%
monounsaturates	65%	Vitamin C	>100%
saturates	20%	Vitamin E	42%
polyunsaturates	15%		

Recommended Red Wines: Chianti Classico, Bulgarian cabernet sauvignon, Cabernet/Tempranillo blends from Penedès.

Meat

∙∙

STEAK AU POIVRE

DELIA SMITH

SERVES 2

In restaurants this is sometimes served swimming in a sickly cream and brandy sauce. Personally I think the combined flavours of the peppercorns and the steak need nothing else but a glass of wine to rinse out the pan at the end.

2 entrecôte (sirloin) steaks, or you could use rump steak if you prefer, weighing 175-225 g (6-8 oz) each
2 heaped teaspoons whole black peppercorns

2 tablespoons olive oil
1 clove garlic, crushed
150 ml (5 fl oz) red wine
salt

First crush the peppercorns very coarsely with a pestle and mortar (or use the back of a tablespoon on a flat surface). Pour the olive oil into a shallow dish, add the crushed garlic, then coat each steak with the oil and press the crushed peppercorns onto both sides of each steak. Then leave them to soak up the flavour in the dish, covered in a cool place for several hours – turning them over once in that time.

When you're ready to cook, pre-heat a thick-based frying-pan (without any fat in it) and when it's very hot sear the steaks quickly on both sides. Then turn down the heat and finish cooking them according to how you like them (a medium-rare entrecôte will take about 6 minutes and should be turned several times during the cooking). One minute before the end of the cooking time pour in the wine, let it bubble, reduce and become syrupy. Then sprinkle a little salt over the steaks and serve immediately with the reduced wine spooned over. These are delicious served with Gratin Dauphinois or jacket potatoes and a green salad.

NUTRITIONAL INFORMATION			
One serving *Steak au Poivre* with a jacket potato and a green salad with 1 teaspoon of vinaigrette			
Calories	911	Protein	19%
Fat	43%	Carbohydrate	33%
of which:		Vitamin A	4%
monounsaturates	40%	Vitamin C	>100%
saturates	33%	Vitamin E	>100%
polyunsaturates	27%		

Recommended Red Wines: Bandol, Fronsac, Blaye, Bordeaux Premières Côtes, Corbières, Argentine cabernet sauvignon.

AGNEAU AUX HERBES

Lamb with Herbs and Garlic

MIREILLE JOHNSTON

SERVES 4

Fontvieille is a pretty village near Arles. Nearby are fragrant fields of rosemary and thyme, Daudet's windmill, sheep and goats roaming on terraced pastures, Roman arenas and olive groves. The village houses have long, narrow, wooden shutters and rust-coloured tiles; the little village square, with its green iron tables and chairs, is sheltered by huge plane trees. It is inland Provence at its best and everybody seems to follow the lizard's advice engraved on fountains and sundials all around: 'I sip life as I sip the sun, by small gulps. Time passes too fast, perhaps it will rain tomorrow.' Taking the time to enjoy life is a priority.

In the centre of the village is a pretty restaurant situated in a disused oil mill and built around a lovely Provençal garden. It is called La Regalido, the Provençal word for the log of wood which is added to the fire as a welcome when guests arrive. Hospitality, warmth and pleasure in all the good things of the land were all present as we entered the kitchen of La Regalido that morning. There was a big bundle of freshly gathered thyme sprinkled with blue blossoms, piles of fresh vegetables, a stack of flat vegetable omelettes ready to be made into an omelette and Monsieur Jean-Pierre Michel was talking to me about olives and describing how local bakers used to crack the stones and place them in the bottom of their ovens to flavour their breads. When the *Agneau aux Herbes* arrived I truly felt like a pampered lizard. As you will see yourself it is very easy to prepare, but the meat must be chosen carefully.

4 thick lamb leg steaks or cutlets
1 teaspoon finely chopped fresh rosemary
1 tablespoon chopped fresh thyme
3½ tablespoons olive oil

16 garlic cloves
40 g (1½ oz) unsalted butter
salt and freshly ground black pepper

Place the lamb in a dish. Sprinkle over half of the thyme and rosemary and 1 tablespoon of olive oil. Turn the lamb over and sprinkle with the remaining herbs and another tablespoon of olive oil. Cover and leave to marinate for about 2 hours.

Thread the garlic cloves on to 4 wooden cocktail sticks. Heat 1½ tablespoons of olive oil and half the butter in a heavy-based frying-pan. When it is very hot, add the lamb and cook quickly for about 3 minutes, turning frequently until evenly browned on all sides. Lower the heat to moderate. Sprinkle the lamb with salt and pepper, and add the remaining butter to the pan. When it begins to sizzle add the garlic cloves and cook until tender and evenly browned.

Transfer the lamb and garlic to 1 large, or 4 individual, warm plates and pour over the cooking juices.

NUTRITIONAL INFORMATION		
One serving *Agneau aux Herbes* (without the juices poured over) with a half serving of ratatouille and a third of a baguette		
Calories	811	Protein	18%
Fat	43%	Carbohydrate	39%
of which:		Vitamin A	33%
monounsaturates	46%	Vitamin C	>100%
saturates	44%	Vitamin E	24%
polyunsaturates	10%		

Recommended Red Wines: Barbaresco, Tempranillo, Bandol, Coonawarra cabernet sauvignon, Barolo, Argentine cabernet sauvignon.

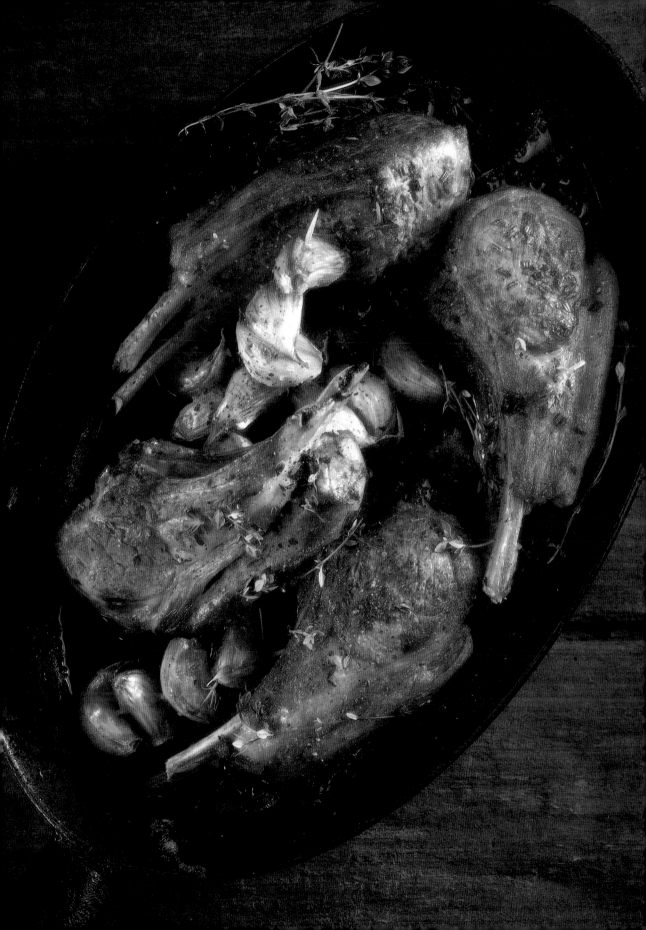

BEEF IN BEER

DELIA SMITH

SERVES 4-6

This is an old Flemish recipe often known by its original name *Carbonnade de Boeuf à la Flamande.* Sometimes large baked croûtons sprinkled with grated cheese are arranged on the top of the cooked beef and the dish is then popped under the grill until the cheese is bubbling. Whether you do this or not, this recipe has a beautiful rich sauce and is one of my firm favourites.

900 g (2 lb) chuck steak, cut into 5 cm
(2 inch) squares
1 tablespoon olive oil
350 g (12 oz) onions, peeled, sliced in
quarters then separated into layers
1 well heaped tablespoon plain flour
425 ml (15 fl oz) light ale

1 sprig fresh thyme, or ½ teaspoon
dried thyme
1 bay leaf
1 fat clove garlic, crushed
salt and freshly milled black pepper

Pre-heat the oven to gas mark 1, 140°C, 275°F.

Heat the oil in a large flameproof casserole until sizzling hot then sear the meat in it - just a few pieces at a time - till they become a dark mahogany brown all over. As the pieces brown, remove them to a plate, then add the onions to the casserole and, with the heat still high, toss them around until brown at the edges. Now return the meat to the casserole together with any juices. Add the flour, turn the heat down, and using a wooden spoon stir it around to soak up all the juices. It will look rather stodgy and unattractive at this stage but that's quite normal.

Next gradually stir in the light ale and, whilst everything *slowly* comes up to simmering point, add the thyme, bay leaf, crushed garlic, and some salt and freshly milled black pepper.

As soon as it begins to simmer, stir thoroughly, put on a tight-fitting lid and transfer the casserole to the middle shelf of the oven.

Cook at a gentle simmer for 2½ hours. Don't take the lid off and have a taste halfway through because, early on, the beer hasn't had time to develop into a delicious sauce; the beautiful aroma will make you very hungry, but please leave it alone!

Note

If you want to serve this in the traditional Flemish way, top with croûtons covered with grated cheese. Just place these on top of the meat with the cheese and brown under the grill. Mashed potatoes and red cabbage are good with this.

NUTRITIONAL INFORMATION			
One serving *Beef in Beer* with mashed potato and red cabbage			
Calories	817	Protein	22%
Fat	46%	Carbohydrate	30%
of which:		Alcohol	2%
monounsaturates	44%	Vitamin A	55%
saturates	50%	Vitamin C	>100%
polyunsaturates	6%	Vitamin E	32%

Recommended Red Wines: Corbières, Gigondas, Washington State cabernet sauvignon, Mexican cabernet sauvignon, Rioja, Barossa Valley Shiraz from Australia.

Marinated Pork with Coriander

Delia Smith

SERVES 3

The Greeks call this traditional dish *Afelia*. If you have time to leave the meat to steep overnight and for the flavours to develop so much the better.

1 pork fillet, cut into bite-sized cubes
3 tablespoons olive oil
juice of 1 lemon
275 ml (10 fl oz) dry white wine (or dry cider)

2 heaped teaspoons coriander seeds, crushed
1 fat clove garlic, crushed
salt and freshly milled black pepper

Place the pieces of pork in a shallow dish and season them with salt and freshly milled pepper. Now pour the oil over the pieces of meat, followed by the juice of the lemon and 2 tablespoons of the white wine. Then sprinkle in the crushed coriander seeds and the garlic, and mix everything together. Cover the dish with a cloth and leave it all to marinate overnight – or as long as possible – stirring now and then.

To cook the pork, melt a little more oil in your largest frying-pan and when it's fairly hot add the cubes of pork and cook them over a medium heat, turning them and keeping them on the move. When they have browned a little, pour in the rest of the white wine, let it bubble and reduce to a syrupy consistency. The pork will take approximately 10-15 minutes to cook altogether. Serve with a little rice and a salad.

NUTRITIONAL INFORMATION			
One serving *Marinated Pork with Coriander* with rice and a green salad with 1 teaspoon of vinaigrette			
Calories	555	Protein	13%
Fat	41%	Carbohydrate	36%
of which:		Alcohol	10%
monounsaturates	64%	Vitamin A	4%
saturates	21%	Vitamin C	38%
polyunsaturates	15%	Vitamin E	24%

Recommended Red Wines: Cahors, Fitou, Barolo, Pinotage, Priorato, Costers del Segre.
White Wines: German Spatlese rieslings at least 10 years old.

MAGRET DE CANARD AU CONFIT D'OIGNONS

Grilled Duck Breast with Caramelized Onion

SOPHIE GRIGSON

SERVES 4

Strictly speaking, *magrets* (or *maigrets*, like the detective) are the breasts of *foie gras* ducks, but the word is now used for any duck breasts, as long as they are nice and plump. They are quick to grill and should remain pink at heart: never overcook to a uniform greyness through and through.

The *confit d'oignons* can be made well ahead of time and is good with any rich meat, be it duck, goose or pork. Served with the duck breasts, and a peppery rocket or watercress salad, it makes for a speedy chic dinner dish.

4 duck breasts
salt and pepper
sunflower or groundnut oil

FOR THE ONION CONFIT
25 g (1 oz) butter

1 tablespoon sunflower or groundnut oil
900 g (2 lb) onions, thinly sliced
50 g (2 oz) caster sugar
2 tablespoons red wine vinegar
2 teaspoons fresh thyme leaves
coarsely ground black pepper

The onion *confit* can be made several days in advance and stored in the refrigerator. Melt the butter with the oil in a wide pan and add the onions. Cook very gently, half-covered, over a low heat, stirring occasionally until the onions are golden and meltingly tender – about 40 minutes. Uncover and stir in the remaining ingredients. Continue cooking for a further 20 minutes or so, stirring frequently, until thick and jammy. Re-heat gently when needed.

Pre-heat the grill thoroughly. Rub salt and pepper into the skin of the duck breasts and grill, skin side to the heat, until well browned. Turn over, brush with oil and grill for a further 5-10 minutes, depending on how well you like them done and how plump the breasts are. Season with salt and pepper, turn off the grill and let the breasts rest for 5 minutes. Slice and arrange on serving plates with a dollop of the warmed onion *confit*.

NUTRITIONAL INFORMATION

One serving *Magret de Canard au Confit d'Oignons* with a green salad and 1 teaspoon of vinaigrette and 2 slices of wholemeal bread

Calories	495	Protein	23%
Fat	35%	Carbohydrate	42%
of which:		Vitamin A	20%
monounsaturates	49%	Vitamin C	52%
saturates	33%	Vitamin E	44%
polyunsaturates	18%		

Recommended Red Wines: Crozes Hermitage, Château Musar, Bandol, Côte Rôtie, Crozes Hermitage, Corbières, Tursan, Californian Zinfandel, Garrafeira.
White Wines: Alsatian Tokay Pinot Gris, South African and New Zealand riesling.

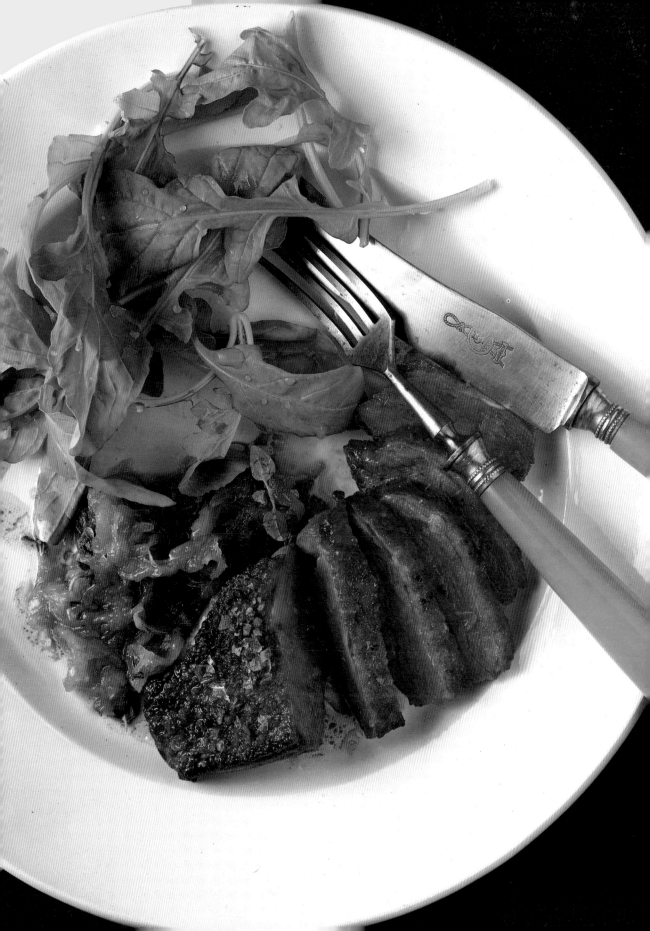

Vegetarian Main Courses

Mixed Vegetables à la Grècque

Delia Smith

Serves 2-4

This is my number one vegetarian dish. It makes an excellent lunch dish with a brown rice salad with a herb vinaigrette, but mostly I serve it as a starter on crisp lettuce leaves with crusty bread to dip into the juices. You can of course vary the vegetables.

6 button onions
50 g (2 oz) dry weight kidney beans,
soaked and cooked
110 g (4 oz) cauliflower, broken into
2.5 cm (1 inch) florets
110 g (4 oz) small to medium mushrooms, halved
4 tablespoons olive oil
1 medium onion, finely chopped
1 fat clove garlic, crushed
2 tablespoons wine vinegar
450 g (1 lb) tomatoes, skinned and quartered, or
400 g (14 oz) tin Italian tomatoes

1 teaspoon dried oregano
1 heaped teaspoon whole coriander seeds, crushed
8 black peppercorns, lightly crushed
juice of 1 medium lemon
55 ml (2 fl oz) water, mixed with 1 heaped teaspoon
tomato purée
salt and freshly milled black pepper

To Serve
2 tablespoons chopped fresh parsley
2 spring onions (including green tops),
finely chopped

Heat 2 tablespoons of the olive oil in a heavy-based pan and soften the onion for 5 minutes. Then add the garlic, wine vinegar, tomatoes, oregano, coriander, peppercorns, lemon juice, water and tomato purée, and some salt. Bring to the boil and stir in the button onions. Now cover the pan and simmer for 20 minutes.

Then add the cooked and drained beans, the cauliflower and mushrooms, cover the pan again and simmer for a further 20 minutes, stirring the vegetables round once or twice during the cooking time. After 20 minutes test the vegetables with a skewer; they should be tender but still firm. Taste and check the seasoning.

Pour the contents of the pan into a shallow dish and leave to cool. I think this dish is best left overnight but a few hours will do. To serve, sprinkle the vegetables with the rest of the olive oil, then scatter the chopped parsley and spring onions on top.

Recommended Red Wines: Moroccan Red, Ribatejo.

NUTRITIONAL INFORMATION			
One serving *Mixed Vegetables à la Grècque* with a green salad with 1 teaspoon of vinaigrette and 2 slices of crusty bread			
Calories	487	Protein	11%
Fat	50%	Carbohydrate	39%
of which:		Vitamin A	48%
monounsaturates	68%	Vitamin C	>100%
saturates	16%	Vitamin E	90%
polyunsaturates	16%		

FAGIOLI ALL'UCCELLETTO

Classic Tuscan Bean Stew

VALENTINA HARRIS

SERVES 6

The Tuscans have been famous as bean eaters for centuries and many recipes for cooking these delicious pulses have originated from the region. The dishes do require fresh beans for the best results, but I think the dried variety works rather well too. This dish is excellent both as an antipasto and an accompaniment.

1.5 kg (3¼ lb) dried haricot, kidney, cannellini or butter beans, soaked overnight in cold water, or canned beans, drained
100 ml (3½ fl oz) best-quality Tuscan olive oil
4 fresh sage leaves or ¼ teaspoon dried sage

2 cloves garlic, peeled
salt and pepper
450 g (1 lb) canned tomatoes, de-seeded and chopped

If using dried beans, drain them and rinse thoroughly in cold water. Put them in a saucepan and cover with fresh cold water. Bring to the boil, boil fast for 5 minutes, drain, rinse and return to the pan. Cover again with fresh cold water, return to the boil and simmer for about 1 hour or until tender - the cooking time will vary according to the type of bean.

Heat the oil in another pan and add the sage, garlic and a large pinch of pepper. Fry for about 5 minutes or until the garlic is golden. Drain the cooked beans and add them to the sage and garlic. If using canned beans, add them at this point also. Stir together and add the tomatoes and their juice. Season to taste with salt and pepper and cover. Simmer slowly for about 20 minutes, making sure the end result is not too dry

– add a little water during cooking if necessary.

NUTRITIONAL INFORMATION			
One serving *Fagioli all Uccelletto* with 2 slices of whole-meal bread			
Calories	473	Protein	17%
Fat	36%	Carbohydrate	47%
of which:		Vitamin A	6%
monounsaturates	68%	Vitamin C	37%
saturates	16%	Vitamin E	54%
polyunsaturates	16%		

Recommended Red Wines: Copertino, Chilean Merlot, Washington State Merlot.

Frittata di Prezzemolo e Basilico

Parsley and Basil Omelette

Valentina Harris

Serves 2

This is a recipe from Puglia, typically simple and delicious. I love to take slices of these omelettes on picnics, to be eaten cold with crusty bread and fresh tomatoes.

4 large free-range eggs
1 handful fresh parsley
1 handful fresh basil

salt and pepper
2 tablespoons milk
4 tablespoons olive oil

Beat the eggs lightly. Remove the leaves from the herbs, wash them and dry them, then tear them up with your fingers. Mix the leaves into the eggs and add salt, pepper and milk.

Heat the olive oil in a heavy-bottomed omelette pan until just beginning to smoke, then tip in the egg mixture. Smooth it out flat with the back of a spoon and cook it on one side for about 5 minutes or until golden. Turn it over on to a lid or large platter, then slide it back into the pan. Cook for a further 3 minutes, transfer to a serving dish and serve hot or cold.

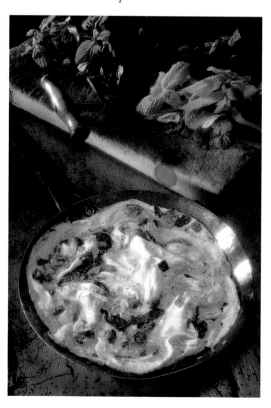

NUTRITIONAL INFORMATION			
One serving *Frittata di Prezzemolo e Basilico* with 2 tomatoes and half a baguette			
Calories	676	Protein	14%
Fat	59%	Carbohydrate	27%
of which:		Vitamin A	55%
monounsaturates	66%	Vitamin C	66%
saturates	21%	Vitamin E	70%
polyunsaturates	13%		

Recommended Red Wines: Chianti Classico, Californian Zinfandel, Copertino, Cabernet/Tempranillo blends.

Above: Frittata Di Prezzemolo E Basilico
Right: Pissaladière (*page 124*)

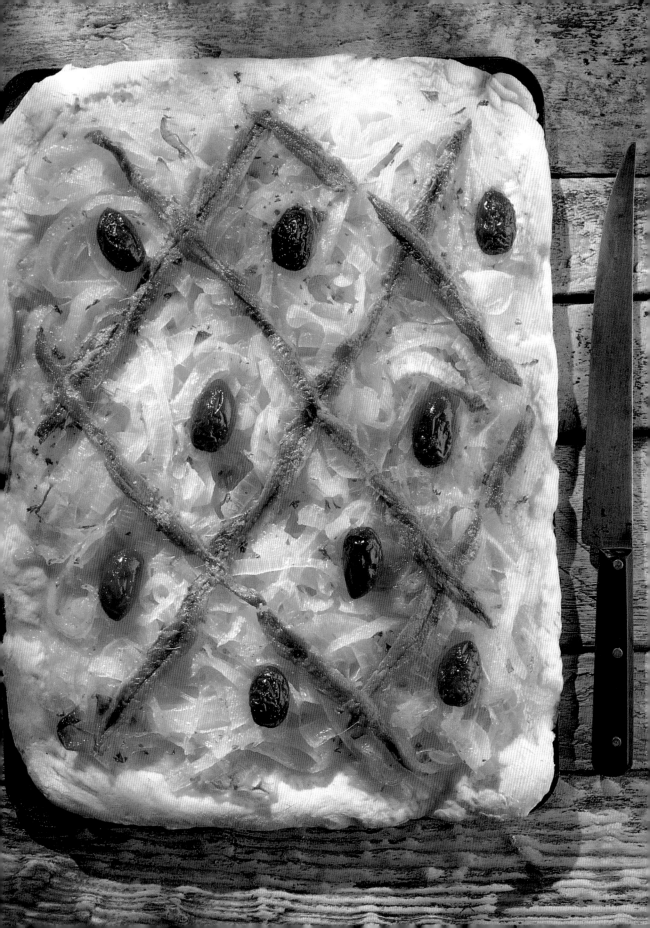

PISSALADIÈRE

Onion Tart

CLAUDIA RODEN

SERVES 6

This famous onion tart of Nice derives its name from the anchovy paste, *pissala*, which used to be brushed on it. Now the traditional anchovy garnish is more often absent while the thick onion filling has become even thicker. I like to use the smaller quantity of onion given but the Niçois prefer the larger amount.

FOR THE DOUGH
250 g (8 oz) plain flour
1 egg, beaten
¾ teaspoon salt
15 g (½ oz) fresh yeast, or 1½ teaspoons
dried yeast
¼ teaspoon sugar
75 ml (3 fl oz) warm water
A few drops of olive oil

FOR THE FILLING
1-2 kg (2-4 lb) onions, thinly sliced
3-4 tablespoons olive oil
salt and pepper
2 teaspoons mixed fresh herbs such as basil, thyme
and rosemary, chopped
12 or more anchovy fillets
a few black olives, stoned and halved

To make the bread dough, sift the flour into a bowl and make a well in the centre. Put the beaten egg and salt in the well. Put the yeast, sugar and water in a bowl and leave it until it froths. Then gradually stir the yeast mixture into the flour, mixing it in with your fingers to form a ball of soft dough. Add a little flour if it is too sticky and knead well with your hands for 10 minutes or until the dough is smooth and elastic. Pour a drop or two of olive oil on the dough and turn it in your hands so that it becomes lightly oiled all over. Cover with a damp cloth and leave to rise in a warm place for an hour or until it doubles in bulk.

While the dough is rising make the filling. Cook the onions in the olive oil in a covered pan on a very low flame, stirring occasionally, for 40 minutes or until they are very soft. Add the salt, pepper and herbs and continue to cook for a few minutes longer. Cut the anchovy fillets in half lengthways.

Pre-heat the oven to gas mark 5, 190°C, 375°F. Grease a pie plate or flan dish about 35 cm (14 in)

in diameter with oil. Punch the dough down, knead it lightly and press it into the pie pan with the palms of your hands. Spread the onion mixture over the dough and make a lattice pattern of anchovy fillets on top. Put half an olive in the middle of each square. Let the dough rise again for 10-15 minutes, then bake for 25-30 minutes or until the bread base is cooked. Serve hot.

NUTRITIONAL INFORMATION			
One serving *Pissaladière* with a green salad and 1 teaspoon of vinaigrette			
Calories	397	Protein	10%
Fat	39%	Carbohydrate	51%
of which:		Vitamin A	10%
monounsaturates	69%	Vitamin C	57%
saturates	16%	Vitamin E	38%
polyunsaturates	15%		

Recommended Red Wines: Rasteau, Moroccan red, Californian Zinfandel.

Pasta, Rice and Pulses

Pasta alla Norma

Sicilian Pasta with Aubergines

Claudia Roden

SERVES 4

On weekends the Sicilian seaside is packed with people from the towns installed table to table on the beaches and in the woods. If you pass between the tables you can see the pasta sauces bubbling over primus stoves. This one was offered to us when we looked into a large saucepan and it was wonderful.

400 g (14 oz) aubergines
salt
1 medium onion, finely chopped
2 tablespoons olive oil
2 garlic cloves, finely chopped
350 g (12 oz) ripe tomatoes, peeled and chopped
black pepper

1 teaspoon sugar (optional)
a few basil leaves, coarsely chopped, or torn, or finely chopped parsley
sunflower or olive oil for frying
400 g (14 oz) spaghetti or rigatoni
40 g (1½ oz) salty Ricotta or Provolone, grated

Dice the aubergines, salt them and leave them for about an hour to disgorge their juices.

To make the sauce, fry the onion in oil till golden. Add the garlic and, when the aroma rises, add the tomatoes, salt and pepper and a little sugar, if using. Cook for 15 minutes or until the tomatoes are soft and the juice reduced, then add the basil.

Wash and dry the aubergines and fry in hot oil until lightly browned and tender, then drain on kitchen paper and add to the sauce. Cook the pasta until *al dente*, drain quickly and mix with the sauce. Stir in the cheese and serve.

NUTRITIONAL INFORMATION			
One serving *Pasta alla Norma* with a green salad and 1 teaspoon of vinaigrette and 2 slices of wholemeal bread			
Calories	453	Protein	12%
Fat	42%	Carbohydrate	46%
of which:		Vitamin A	34%
monounsaturates	61%	Vitamin C	>100%
saturates	24%	Vitamin E	48%
polyunsaturates	15%		

Recommended Red Wines: Chianti, Barbaresco, Bulgarian cabernet sauvignon, Chilean Merlot.

FUSILLI WITH SMOKED TROUT, ROCKET AND BASIL

SOPHIE GRIGSON

SERVES 4

This dish takes just minutes to make – the rocket, basil and smoked fish cooking instantly in the heat of the pasta.

1 handful of rocket leaves
400 g (14 oz) fusilli or other pasta shapes
6 tablespoons olive oil
juice of ½ lemon
2 cloves garlic, peeled and crushed

salt and freshly ground black pepper
12 large fresh basil leaves, shredded
175 g (6 oz) sliced smoked trout,
cut into short thin strips

I f the rocket leaves are fairly large, tear them up roughly. If they are tiny, 5 cm (2 inches) or so in length, tear or snip them in half. Prepare all the remaining ingredients.

Cook the fusilli in a large pan of lightly salted water until just *al dente*. Drain well and return to the pan, set over a low heat. Toss in the olive oil, lemon juice, garlic, a little salt and plenty of pepper. Stir for a couple of seconds, then add the rocket and basil and toss again to mix evenly. Draw off the heat and finally toss in the trout. Serve immediately.

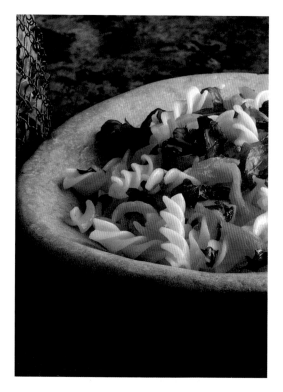

NUTRITIONAL INFORMATION			
One serving *Fusilli with Smoked Trout , Rocket and Basil* with 2 slices of wholemeal bread			
Calories	742	Protein	15%
Fat	35%	Carbohydrate	50%
of which:		Vitamin A	41%
monounsaturates	65%	Vitamin C	>100%
saturates	18%	Vitamin E	36%
polyunsaturates	17%		

Recommended Red Wines: Chilled Copertino, Kekfrancos, Alentejo, young Tempranillo.
White Wines: Moselle riesling, New Zealand sauvignon blanc.

Above: FUSILLI WITH SMOKED TROUT, ROCKET AND BASIL
Right: RISOTTO CON GAMBERETTI (*page 128*)

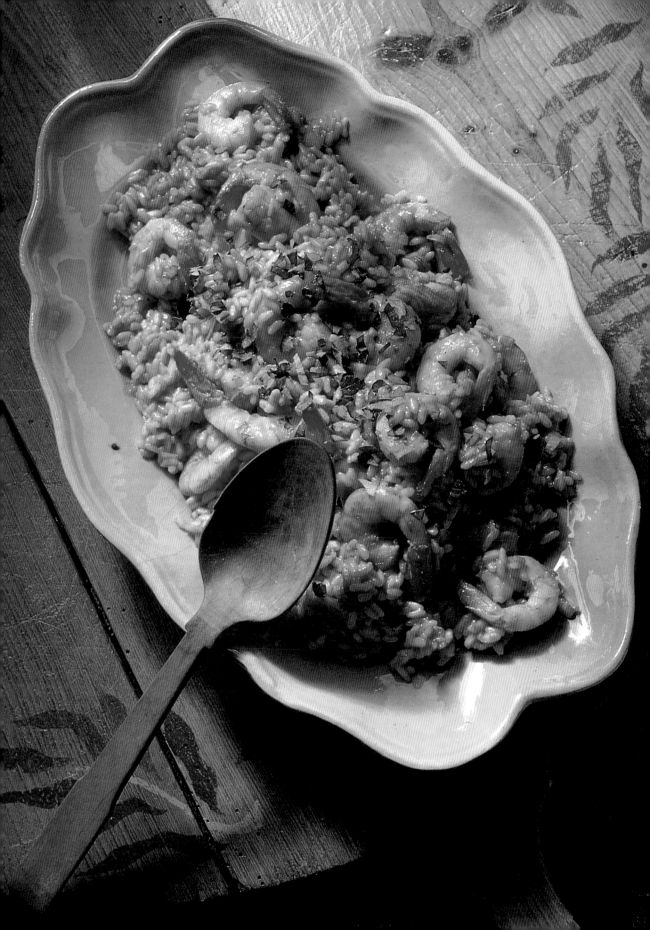

RISOTTO CON GAMBERETTI

Risotto with Prawns

VALENTINA HARRIS

SERVES 6

Raw prawns are essential for this dish as they give it extra sweetness and fishy flavour. Order them in advance from your fishmonger who should be able to get them for you if he has enough notice. It makes a marvellous dinner or luncheon-party dish.

750 g (1 lb 10 oz) raw prawns
1 small onion, peeled and finely chopped
1 clove garlic, peeled and finely chopped
1 small carrot, finely chopped
½ stick celery, chopped
4 tablespoons olive oil
4 tablespoons dry white wine
1 litre (1¾ pints) cold water

salt and freshly ground black pepper
2 tablespoons unsalted butter
1 shallot, peeled and thinly sliced
2 tablespoons brandy
1 tablespoon tomato purée
500 g (1 lb 2 oz) risotto rice
50 g (2 oz) Parmesan cheese, freshly grated

Remove the heads and legs from the prawns, extract the tails and set them aside. Put all the shells and heads into a saucepan with the onion, garlic, carrot, celery and 3 tablespoons of oil and fry gently for about 5 minutes. Add the wine and boil off the alcohol for 2 minutes then add the water and season to taste with salt and pepper. Bring to the boil, cover and leave to simmer gently. In a separate saucepan, heat the remaining oil with the butter and fry the shallot very gently for about 5 minutes. Add the prawn tails and cook for 5 minutes. Pour on the brandy and boil off the alcohol for 2 minutes. Stir in the tomato purée. Add the rice all in one go and stir it around until it is heated through and shining. Then add the first ladleful of stock from the prawn shells. Stir until the stock has been absorbed, then add more. Always add small amounts and always wait for the rice to absorb the stock before you add any more. Continue this for about 20 minutes until the rice is swollen but still firm in the middle. Stir in the remaining butter and the Parmesan. Remove from the heat, cover and leave to stand for about 3 minutes. Transfer to a warmed serving platter and serve at once.

NUTRITIONAL INFORMATION			
One serving *Risotto Con Gamberetti*			
Calories	591	Protein	14%
Fat	40%	Carbohydrate	43%
of which:		Alcohol	3%
monounsaturates	51%	Vitamin A	46%
saturates	37%	Vitamin C	11%
polyunsaturates	12%	Vitamin E	18%

Recommended Red Wines: Barolo, Chianti, Copertino.
White Wines: chardonnays from Puglia in Italy, Australian Hunter Valley chardonnays.

Vegetable Side Dishes

LEEKS VINAIGRETTE

SOPHIE GRIGSON

SERVES 4

Sometimes known as Poor Man's Asparagus, *Leeks Vinaigrette* is a fine dish in its own right. It makes a wonderful first course, too, when served with good bread to mop up the juices. When I can get them, I use slim baby leeks, more like large spring onions, allowing 3-4 per person, but larger leeks work almost as well. Do be careful not to overcook the leeks, and to drain them really thoroughly. Slimy waterlogged leeks are no fun.

8 medium leeks, trimmed
1 tablespoon white wine vinegar
½ teaspoon Dijon mustard
salt and freshly ground black pepper

4-5 tablespoons olive oil
1 hard-boiled egg, finely chopped
1 tablespoon chopped fresh parsley

Boil or steam the leeks until just tender. While they are cooking make the vinaigrette: whisk the vinegar with the mustard, salt and pepper. Gradually whisk in the olive oil, a tablespoon at a time. Taste and adjust seasoning. Drain the leeks thoroughly then, while still hot, place in a shallow dish and spoon over the vinaigrette. Leave to cool, then scatter with the chopped egg and parsley.

NUTRITIONAL INFORMATION			
One serving *Leeks Vinaigrette* with 2 slices of wholemeal bread			
Calories	385	Protein	16%
Fat	47%	Carbohydrate	37%
of which:		Vitamin A	>100%
monounsaturates	62%	Vitamin C	>100%
saturates	18%	Vitamin E	>100%
polyunsaturates	20%		

STOVED POTATOES WITH GARLIC AND CORIANDER

SOPHIE GRIGSON

SERVES 3-4

Slowly cooked in olive oil, stoved potatoes are meltingly tender. The whole cloves of garlic not only give flavour, but soften and mellow to a mild sweetness. This is a lovely way to cook both new and old potatoes.

450 g (1 lb) new potatoes or waxier main-crop potatoes (e.g. Cara)
1 head of garlic

salt and freshly ground black pepper
3 tablespoons olive oil
2 tablespoons chopped fresh coriander

If the new potatoes are very small, leave them as they are. With medium-sized ones, cut in half or quarters. The aim is to get all the chunks about the same size so that they cook evenly. If using main-crop potatoes peel and cut into 2.5-4 cm (1-1½ inch) chunks. Separate all the cloves of garlic and peel, but leave whole.

Put the potatoes and garlic into a heavy frying-pan in a single layer. Don't try to force them in too tightly, because you have to be able to turn them. If you've got a few bits too many, then leave them out. Season with salt and pepper, then add 6 tablespoons of water. Drizzle over the olive oil.

Cook, covered, over a low heat for 40 minutes, shaking the pan and stirring occasionally, until the potatoes and garlic are very tender and patched with brown. By then the water should have been absorbed. If not, uncover the pan and boil it off. Once they are done, sprinkle over the coriander and serve.

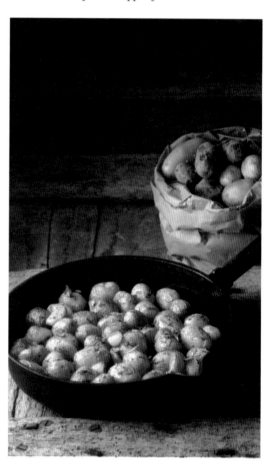

NUTRITIONAL INFORMATION			
One serving *Stoved Potatoes with Garlic and Coriander*			
Calories	181	Protein	5%
Fat	57%	Carbohydrate	38%
of which:		Vitamin A	3%
monounsaturates	71%	Vitamin C	92%
saturates	16%	Vitamin E	14%
polyunsaturates	13%		

Above: STOVED POTATOES WITH GARLIC AND CORIANDER
Right: HENRI FONTIN'S RATATOUILLE (*page 132*)

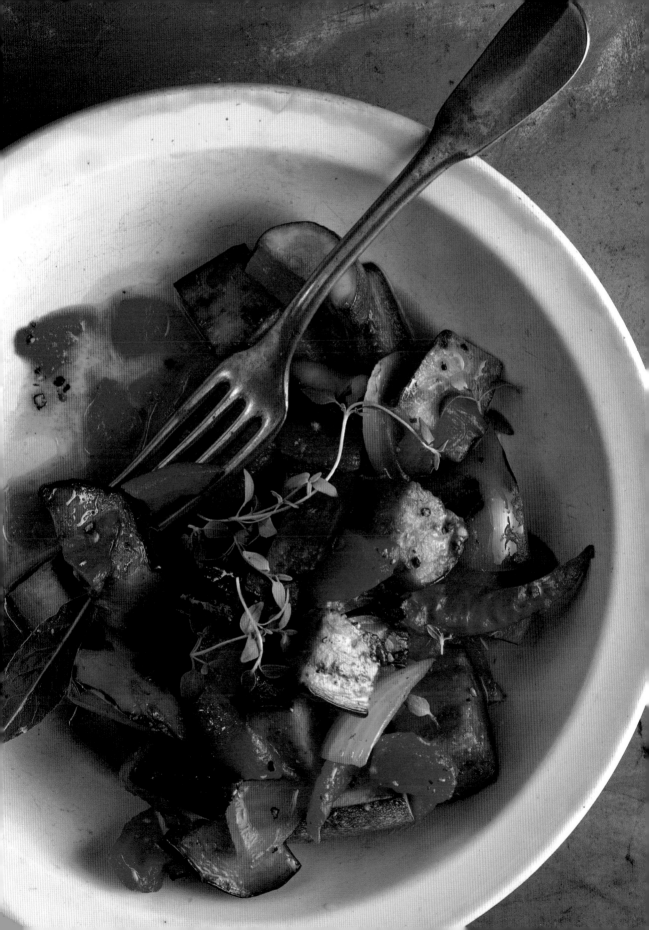

Henri Fontin's Ratatouille

Claudia Roden

SERVES 6

A ratatouille can be served hot or cold, as a side dish, an hors d'oeuvre or a main dish. In Nice all the vegetables are fried separately. As this takes time and requires many pans it is worth making a large amount to eat over several days. The proportions of vegetables vary; the following are the preference of Henri Fontin who gives Provençal cookery lessons in the youth hostel he runs in Séguret near Avignon.

750g (1½lb) aubergines
500g (1 lb) courgettes
2 green peppers
1 large Spanish onion, peeled
olive oil
salt and pepper

2 large beef tomatoes, peeled and de-seeded
1 teaspoon fresh thyme
2 bay leaves
¼-½ teaspoon cayenne pepper, or
1 small dried chilli

Cut the vegetables into 1-1.5 cm (½-¾ in) pieces. Fry the first 4 vegetables separately. Fry the courgettes, peppers and onion in 2 or more tablespoons of oil each very gently on low heat, until they are cooked *al dente* - tender but still firm. The aubergines will need more oil and it must be hot to begin with to seal them. Cook them until they are very soft. Add salt and pepper to taste. Combine the cooked vegetables with the tomatoes, herbs and cayenne pepper or chilli for 15 minutes more over medium heat, stirring constantly.

Variations

Fry 5 finely chopped garlic cloves, add 750 g (1½ lb) of peeled, deseeded and chopped tomatoes and cook until they are reduced to a thick sauce. Add this to the vegetables instead of the two tomatoes.

Caponata is a Sicilian relative of ratatouille. Make it like ratatouille but without peppers and courgettes. Add 3 celery stalks, coarsely chopped, a handful of pitted green olives and 2 tablespoons of capers. Give it a sweet and sour taste with 4 tablespoons wine vinegar, 1 tablespoon sugar and, if you like, 1-2 tablespoons of cocoa powder. Garnish with toasted, chopped almonds and chopped parsley.

NUTRITIONAL INFORMATION			
One serving *Henri Fontin's Ratatouille*			
Calories	78	Protein	18%
Fat	41%	Carbohydrate	41%
of which:		Vitamin A	32%
monounsaturates	55%	Vitamin C	>100%
saturates	18%	Vitamin E	18%
polyunsaturates	27%		

Broccoli with Chilli and Parmesan

Sophie Grigson

Serves 4

This is a quick way to dress up cooked broccoli with a dash of fire. Spiked with chilli and garlic, melting slivers of Parmesan on top, it's a nifty way to transform broccoli into something special.

750 g (1½ lb) broccoli
salt
3 tablespoons olive oil
¼-½ teaspoon chilli flakes

2-3 cloves garlic, peeled and finely chopped
15 g (½ oz) Parmesan cheese, cut into
paper-thin slivers

Separate the broccoli florets from the stalks. Slice the stalks about 1 cm (½ inch) thick. Drop the stalks into a pan of lightly salted boiling water. Simmer for 2 minutes, then add the florets and cook for a further 2-3 minutes until almost but not quite done. Drain, run under the cold tap to refresh then leave to drain completely and pat dry on kitchen paper.

Heat the oil in a wide frying-pan, and add the chilli and garlic. Cook over a low heat for about 1 minute, then add the broccoli. Raise the heat a little and stir and fry for 4-5 minutes until the broccoli is piping hot. Tip into a serving dish and scatter over the Parmesan. Serve at once.

NUTRITIONAL INFORMATION			
One serving *Broccoli with Chilli and Parmesan*			
Calories	167	Protein	19%
Fat	75%	Carbohydrate	6%
of which:		Vitamin A	33%
monounsaturates	64%	Vitamin C	>100%
saturates	20%	Vitamin E	54%
polyunsaturates	16%		

Salads

Insalata Caprese

Capri Salad

Valentina Harris

Serves 4

Everybody's favourite! My friend Vera Oliviero and I prepared this on the terrace of her glorious villa overlooking the bay of Positano. You are unlikely to find the delicious pink tomatoes that she used anywhere other than in the Positano area – apparently the volcanic soil gives them their strange colour and texture. They were the most delicious tomatoes I have ever eaten. As a substitute, use beef or marmande tomatoes, or organically grown tomatoes – they taste more like Italian ones! As for Vera's husband Nello's amazing basil, it was exceptionally perfumed! You must be sure to use really fresh Mozzarella in this recipe. Press it gently between your finger and thumb: if it's fresh it should be very soft and wet. The salad was originally created on the island of Capri, which is how it got its name.

2-3 large tomatoes
150 g (5 oz) very fresh Mozzarella cheese
1 large handful fresh basil leaves, torn and whole

olive oil
salt and pepper

Wash the tomatoes and cut them into thickish slices. Slice the mozzarella into similar-shaped pieces.

Arrange the tomato and mozzarella slices alternately on a platter, working round the edges in a circle. Fill the centre if you have enough slices left over.

Scatter with the basil, then dress with oil and salt and pepper to taste. Serve at once, or after no more than 30 minutes.

Nutritional Information			
One serving *Insalata Caprese*			
Calories	253	Protein	15%
Fat	82%	Carbohydrate	3%
of which:		Vitamin A	43%
monounsaturates	52%	Vitamin C	61%
saturates	41%	Vitamin E	32%
polyunsaturates	7%		

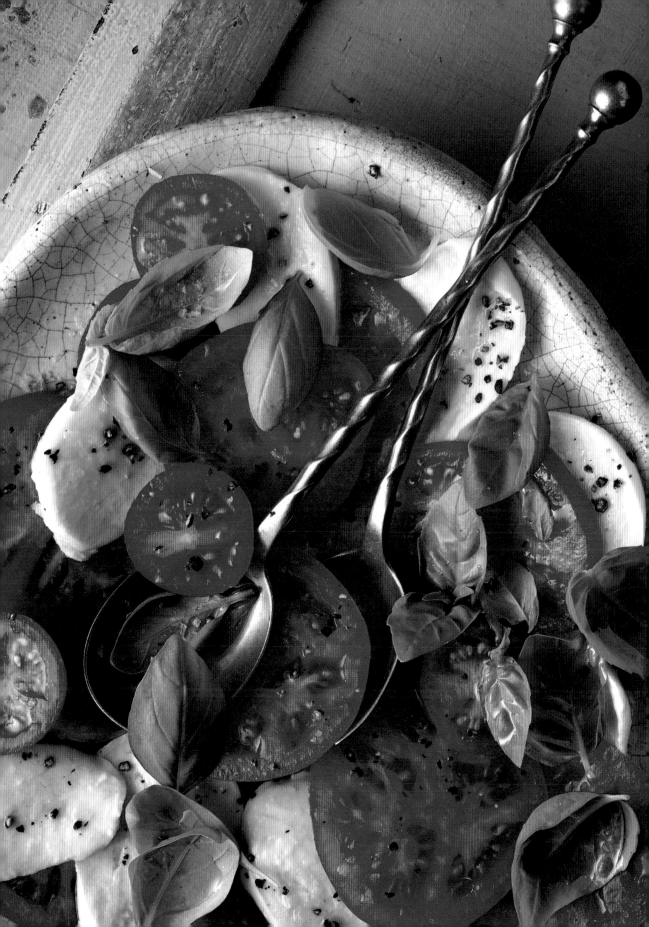

CAESAR SALAD

SOPHIE GRIGSON

SERVES 6

There are many recipes for this most famous of salads, invented in the 1920s by Caesar Cardini at his restaurant in Tijuana, Mexico. The original didn't include anchovies, but they often creep in none the less. The final preparation (which I've simplified a little) can be done discreetly in the kitchen, or more dramatically at the dinner table. If you choose to perform publicly, make sure you have a very large bowl, so that you don't shower your audience with lettuce.

2 cos lettuces
3 slices stale white bread, crusts removed, cut into
1-cm (½-inch) cubes
3 cloves garlic
160 ml (5 fl oz) extra virgin olive oil
2 eggs

½ tin anchovy fillets, finely chopped or
½ teaspoon Worcestershire sauce
juice of 1 lemon
salt and freshly ground black pepper
25 g (1 oz) freshly grated Parmesan cheese

In advance: wash and dry the lettuce well. Store in the fridge in a plastic bag until needed. Fry the cubes of bread with the garlic in 5 tablespoons of the olive oil, until golden and crisp. Drain the croûtons on kitchen paper. Put the eggs into a pan, cover with water, and bring to the boil. Boil for 1 minute, then drain and run under the cold tap.

At the last minute: tear the lettuce up into manageable pieces and place in a large salad bowl. Pour over 6 tablespoons of olive oil and toss to coat each leaf. Add anchovies or Worcestershire sauce, croûtons, lemon juice, pepper and a little salt. Toss. Finally break in the eggs, taking care not to get specks of shell into the salad, and scatter with the Parmesan. Toss or turn again to mix evenly. Now, with all the work done, you can serve it.

NUTRITIONAL INFORMATION			
One serving *Caesar Salad*			
Calories	339	Protein	8%
Fat	83%	Carbohydrate	9%
of which:		Vitamin A	18%
monounsaturates	70%	Vitamin C	38%
saturates	18%	Vitamin E	40%
polyunsaturates	12%		

GREEN LEAF SALAD WITH WALNUTS

SOPHIE GRIGSON

SERVES 4

Even supermarkets now sell the rarer nut oils, and a jolly good thing too. A vinaigrette made with nut oil and a scattering of matching toasted nuts gives a simple salad a major lift. Walnuts and walnut oil are excellent, but you might also try toasted hazelnuts or pine kernels with hazelnut oil.

25 g (1 oz) walnut pieces
selection of salad leaves (e.g. cos, frisée, radicchio, batavia, lollo rosso)

FOR THE DRESSING
1 tablespoon red wine vinegar

½-1 clove garlic, peeled and crushed (optional)
salt and freshly ground black pepper
pinch of sugar
3 tablespoons walnut oil and 2 tablespoons sunflower or groundnut oil

Pre-heat the oven to gas mark 6-8, 200-230°C, 400-450°F. Spread the walnut pieces out on a baking sheet and cook for 5-10 minutes, shaking tray occasionally, until the walnuts are patched with dark brown. Tip into a wire sieve and shake to dislodge any papery flakes of skin. Cool.

Wash and dry the salad leaves. Store in a knotted plastic bag in the bottom of the fridge until needed. Either put all dressing ingredients in a screwtop jar and shake well to mix, or whisk the vinegar with the garlic, salt, pepper and sugar and then gradually whisk in the oil. Taste and adjust seasonings.

Just before serving shake the dressing, and pour about half of it (save the rest for another salad) into a salad bowl. Cross salad servers in the bowl, and arrange the leaves on top. Scatter with the walnuts and toss at table.

NUTRITIONAL INFORMATION			
One serving *Green Leaf Salad with Walnuts*			
Calories	133	Protein	4%
Fat	93%	Carbohydrate	3%
of which:		Vitamin A	6%
monounsaturates	32%	Vitamin C	11%
saturates	15%	Vitamin E	64%
polyunsaturates	53%		

ROASTED VEGETABLE COUS-COUS SALAD WITH HARISSA-STYLE DRESSING

DELIA SMITH

SERVES 4 AS A MAIN COURSE OR 8 AS A STARTER

This salad is one of the best vegetarian dishes I've ever served. The combination of goat's cheese and roasted vegetables on a cool bed of cous-cous mixed with salad leaves and a spicy dressing is positively five-star.

450 g (1 lb) cherry tomatoes, skinned
1 small aubergine
2 medium courgettes
1 small red pepper, deseeded and cut into
2.5 cm (1 inch) squares
1 large onion, sliced and cut into 2.5 cm
(1 inch) squares
2 fat cloves garlic, crushed
3 tablespoons extra virgin olive oil
2 tablespoons fresh basil, leaves torn so that they stay
quite visible
salt and freshy milled black pepper
1 small bulb fennel, chopped

FOR THE COUS COUS

275 g (10 oz) medium cous-cous
500 ml (18 fl oz) vegetable stock
110 g (4 oz) firm goat's cheese

salt and freshly milled black pepper

FOR THE SALAD

1 x 75 g (3 oz) packet mixed salad leaves (such as
lettuce, coriander leaves, flat-leaf parsley, rocket)

FOR THE DRESSING

110 ml (4 fl oz) extra virgin olive oil
1 rounded teaspoon cayenne pepper
2 tablespoons ground cumin
2 heaped tablespoons tomato purée
4 tablespoons lime juice (approx. 2 limes)

TO GARNISH

1 tablespoon black onion seeds

Pre-heat the oven to gas mark 9, 240°C, 475°F.

Prepare the aubergine and courgettes ahead of time by cutting them into 2.5 cm (1 inch) dice, leaving the skins on. Then toss the dice in about a level dessertspoon of salt and pack them into a colander with a plate on top and a heavy weight on top of the plate. Leave them on one side for an hour so that some of the bitter juices drain out. After that squeeze out any juices left, and dry the dice thoroughly in a clean cloth.

Now arrange the tomatoes, aubergine, courgettes, peppers and onion in the roasting-tin, sprinkle with the chopped garlic, basil and olive oil, toss everything around in the oil to get a good coating, and season with salt and pepper. Now place the tin on the highest shelf of the oven for 30-40 minutes or until the vegetables are toasted brown at the edges. Remove them to a plate to cool.

When you're ready to assemble the salad, first place the cous-cous in a large, heatproof bowl, then pour the boiling stock over it, add some salt and pepper, stir it with a fork, then leave on one side for 5 minutes, by which time it will have absorbed all the stock and softened.

Meanwhile, cut the cheese into sugar-cube-sized pieces. Make up the dressing by whisking all the ingredients together in a bowl, then pour into a serving jug. To serve the salad, place the cous-cous in a large, wide salad bowl and gently fork in the cubes of cheese along with the roasted vegetables. Next arrange the salad leaves on top and, just before serving, drizzle a little of the dressing over the top followed by a sprinkling of onion seeds and hand the rest of the dressing round separately.

NUTRITIONAL INFORMATION			
One serving *Roasted Vegetable Cous-cous Salad with Harissa-style Dressing*			
Calories	363	Protein	11%
Fat	69%	Carbohydrate	20%
of which:		Vitamin A	61%
monounsaturates	60%	Vitamin C	>100%
saturates	29%	Vitamin E	52%
polyunsaturates	11%		

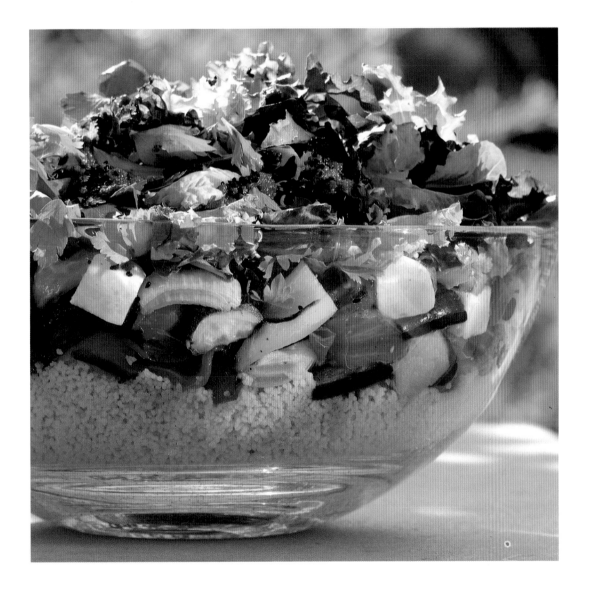

FRENCH BEAN AND BACON SALAD

SOPHIE GRIGSON

SERVES 4

Once a year I teach a children's cookery holiday, and on the last day the children and I have to prepare a meal for 70 people between us. We use whatever vegetables we have to hand to make huge bowls of salad. I gave one group of boys a box of French beans and some bacon, a few vague instructions, and this is what they came up with, though in rather larger quantity. The garlic and Worcestershire sauce were their additions, and are what really make the salad.

450 g (1 lb) French beans
4 rashers streaky bacon
2 tablespoons chopped fresh parsley

FOR THE DRESSING
1 clove garlic, peeled and crushed
½ tablespoon white wine vinegar
1 teaspoon Worcestershire sauce
3 tablespoons olive oil
salt and freshly ground black pepper

To make the dressing, whisk the crushed garlic with the vinegar and Worcestershire sauce. Gradually beat in the olive oil, and add salt and pepper to taste.

Top and tail the beans and cut into 2.5-4 cm (1-1½ inch) lengths. Drop into a pan of boiling salted water and simmer for about 3 minutes or until just tender but retaining a slight crunch. Drain thoroughly and mix with enough of the dressing to coat well. Grill the rashers of bacon until browned then cut into small strips. Toss with the green beans and the parsley. Taste, and adjust seasoning, adding a little extra Worcestershire sauce if necessary. Serve.

NUTRITIONAL INFORMATION			
One serving *French Bean and Bacon Salad*			
Calories	289	Protein	11%
Fat	84%	Carbohydrate	5%
of which:		Vitamin A	22%
monounsaturates	57%	Vitamin C	>100%
saturates	30%	Vitamin E	20%
polyunsaturates	13%		

NIÇOISE SALAD

CLAUDIA RODEN

SERVES 6

Catherine-Hélène Barale, who runs a restaurant in Nice of the same name, is a formidable elderly woman who fiercely upholds Niçois cookery traditions. According to her, the true *salade niçoise* never contains potatoes or any other boiled vegetable. Here, then, is the 'real thing', made with raw vegetables only and including plenty of tomatoes.

10 medium-sized tomatoes, cut in quarters
salt
1 garlic clove
1 large cucumber, peeled and thinly sliced
200 g (7 oz) very young broad beans or
baby artichokes, thinly sliced (optional)
2 green peppers, thinly sliced
6 spring onions, thinly sliced
12 anchovy fillets cut into pieces

a 250 g (8 oz) tin of tuna, flaked
125 g (4 oz) black olives
3 hard-boiled eggs, shelled and thinly sliced

FOR THE DRESSING
90 ml (3½ fl oz) olive oil
2 tablespoons red wine vinegar
6 basil leaves, finely chopped (optional)
salt and pepper

Sprinkle the tomatoes lightly with salt and let their juices drain. Cut the garlic clove in half and rub the inside of a bowl or a large serving dish. Arrange all the ingredients decoratively in the dish. Combine the dressing ingredients, pour over the salad, then serve.

NUTRITIONAL INFORMATION		
One serving *Salade Niçoise*		
Calories	298	Protein	25%
Fat	64%	Carbohydrate	11%
of which:		Vitamin A	37%
monounsaturates	68%	Vitamin C	>100%
saturates	18%	Vitamin E	60%
polyunsaturates	14%		

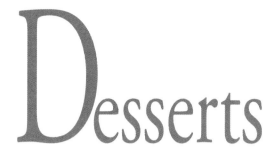

Desserts

Tarte au Citron et à l'Orange

Lemon, Orange and Almond Tart

Mireille Johnston

SERVES 8

Topped with pieces of fruit, *Tarte au Citron* has a refreshing texture and flavour, and the combination of crisp pastry shell and light, sharp custard topped by a layer of orange and lemon pieces covered with marmalade and toasted almonds is irresistible.

FOR THE PASTRY	FOR THE FILLING
175 g (6 oz) plain flour	*3 lemons*
90 g (3½ oz) butter	*2 oranges*
2 egg yolks	*75 g (3 oz) caster sugar*
a pinch of salt	*70 g (2½ oz) unsalted butter*
75 g (3 oz) icing sugar	*2 eggs*
2 tablespoons very cold water	*4 tablespoons sieved orange marmalade*
	25 g (1 oz) flaked almonds
	icing sugar, for dusting

Sift the flour on to the work surface and form a well in the centre. Place the butter, egg yolks, salt, sugar and water in the well and gradually work in the flour using the fingertips to make a soft dough; add a little flour if it is too sticky or add a little water if it is too dry. Form the dough into a ball. Push the dough away from you with the heel of one hand. Gather it up again using a metal palette knife or pastry scraper and repeat for 1-2 minutes. Form into a ball, cover with cling film and chill for 45 minutes.

Pre-heat the oven to gas mark 6, 200°C, 400°F.

Butter a 23 cm (9 in) loose-bottomed flan tin.

Using a rolling pin, flatten the dough, then roll it out into a circle about 27 cm (11 in) in diameter. Fold the dough back over the rolling pin and carefully lift it over the flan tin. Press the dough into the shape of the tin, allowing the excess to hang over the rim. Pass the rolling pin across the top of the rim to cut off the dough neatly. With the thumb of one hand, push the edge of the pastry inwards gently, then, with a finger of the other hand, pinch the pastry pushed up initially to crimp it. Continue around the edge of the pastry shell.

Prick the bottom of the pastry shell with a fork. Place in the fridge for 15-20 minutes.

Lower the oven temperature to gas mark 5, 190°C, 375°F. Line the pastry shell with greaseproof paper, fill with baking beans and place the flan tin on a baking sheet. Bake for 15 minutes until set and lightly browned. Remove the baking beans and greaseproof paper and bake the pastry for a further 5 minutes. Leave to cool.

Grate the rind from one of the lemons and ½ an orange. Squeeze the juice from 2 lemons. Beat together the sugar, butter and orange and lemon rinds until light and fluffy. Gradually beat in the eggs. Slowly stir in the lemon juice.

Peel both oranges and the remaining lemon as you would in order to eat them, then using a sharp knife carefully scrape off the pith. Holding the fruit over a bowl to catch any drips, cut down between the membrane and the fruit to remove the segments. Add any juice collected in the bowl to the butter mixture and spread in the pastry case. Place the lemon and orange segments on top, pressing them down lightly.

Warm the marmalade in a small saucepan over a low heat. Carefully brush over the orange and lemon segments then sprinkle with the almonds. Bake in the oven for 15 minutes. Leave to cool for 10 minutes then transfer to a wire rack to cool completely. Dust with icing sugar just before serving the tart.

NUTRITIONAL INFORMATION			
One serving *Tarte au Citron et à l'Orange*			
Calories	374	Protein	5%
Fat	47%	Carbohydrate	48%
of which:		Vitamin A	45%
monounsaturates	29%	Vitamin C	>100%
saturates	66%	Vitamin E	16%
polyunsaturates	5%		

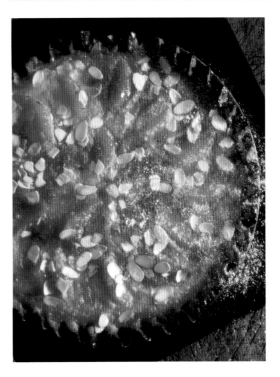

SUFFLÉ DI ALBICOCCHE

Apricot Soufflé

VALENTINA HARRIS

SERVES 6

A lovely hot and light apricot soufflé with almonds, I don't usually serve this with cream, but a scoop of vanilla ice-cream provides an excellent contrast in texture and flavour.

350 g (12 oz) apricots
400 g (14 oz) caster sugar
1 teaspoon vanilla essence
8 egg whites, chilled

2 tablespoons unsalted butter
3 tablespoons ground almonds
2 tablespoons icing sugar, sifted

Pre-heat the oven to gas mark 4, 180°C, 350°F. Put the apricots and sugar into a saucepan and poach the apricots gently until soft. Remove all the stones and sieve the mixture carefully. Leave it to cool completely. Stir in the vanilla essence. Whisk the egg whites until completely stiff and then fold them lightly but thoroughly into the apricot mixture.

Generously butter the base and sides of a 2 litre (3½ pint) soufflé dish and coat with the ground almonds. Pour in the apricot mixture and bake in the centre of the oven for about 35 minutes until well risen and fairly firm. Dust with icing sugar and serve at once.

NUTRITIONAL INFORMATION			
One serving *Sufflé di Albicocche*			
Calories	730	Protein	6%
Fat	19%	Carbohydrate	75%
of which:		Vitamin A	31%
monounsaturates	46%	Vitamin C	26%
saturates	39%	Vitamin E	70%
polyunsaturates	15%		

CRÈME CARAMEL

DELIA SMITH

SERVES 4-6

My husband Michael always makes this at home. It turns out in a pool of lovely dark toffee caramel, and is soft and creamy within. If you are feeling really wicked serve it with some chilled Jersey pouring cream - ecstasy!

150 ml (5 fl oz) milk
275 ml (10 fl oz) single cream
4 large eggs
40 g (1½ oz) soft brown sugar
pure vanilla essence

FOR THE CARAMEL
110g (4 oz) granulated or caster sugar
2 tablespoons water, tap hot

Pre-heat the oven to gas mark 2, 150°C, 300°F.
A 850 ml (1½ pint) soufflé dish.

First make the caramel. Put the granulated (or caster) sugar in a medium-sized saucepan and heat. When the sugar begins to melt, bubble and darken, stir and continue to cook until it has become a uniform liquid syrup, about two or three shades darker than golden syrup. Take the pan off the heat and cautiously add the water – it will splutter and bubble quite considerably but will soon subside. Stir and, when the syrup is once again smooth, quickly pour it into the base of the dish, tipping it around to coat the sides a little.

Now pour the milk and cream into another pan and leave it to heat gently while you whisk together the eggs, brown sugar and a few drops of vanilla essence in a large bowl. Then, when the milk is steaming hot, pour it onto the egg and sugar mixture, whisking until thoroughly blended. Then pour the liquid into the dish and place it in a large roasting tin. Transfer the tin carefully to the oven, then pour hot water into it to surround the dish up to two-thirds in depth. Bake for 1 hour. Cool and chill the crème caramel, until 1 hour before you're ready to serve it. Free the edges by running a knife around before inverting it onto a serving plate.

NUTRITIONAL INFORMATION			
One serving *Crème Caramel*			
Calories	306	Protein	10%
Fat	47%	Carbohydrate	43%
of which:		Vitamin A	55%
monounsaturates	36%	Vitamin C	4%
saturates	58%	Vitamin E	14%
polyunsaturates	6%		

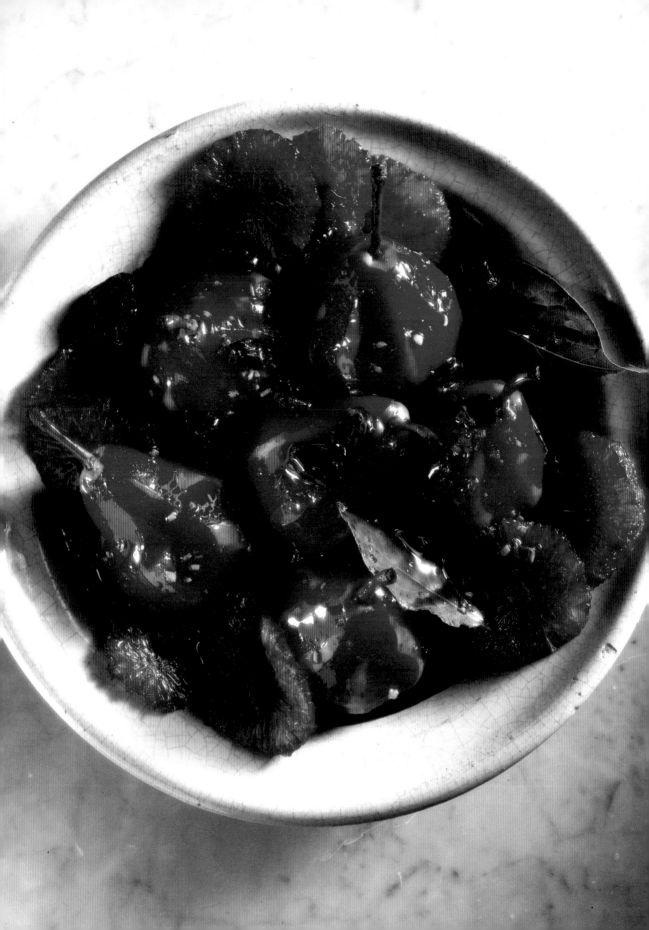

POIRES, PRUNEAUX ET ORANGES AU VIN ROUGE AT AUX EPICES

Pears, Prunes and Oranges Cooked in Red Wine with Spices

MIREILLE JOHNSTON

SERVES 6

100 g (4 oz) plump raisins
6 large prunes, stoned
1 lemon
3 oranges
6 firm but ripe pears with stems
600 ml (1 pint) full-bodied red wine
175 g (6 oz) sugar

4 teaspoons black peppercorns
a pinch of freshly grated nutmeg
1 cinnamon stick
1 teaspoon coriander seeds
1 clove
2 bay leaves
1 tablespoon finely chopped fresh ginger

Place the raisins and prunes in a bowl, pour over boiling water and leave for 1-2 hours. Using a potato peeler, pare 2 large strips of rind from the lemon and 1 of the oranges, then squeeze the juice from the lemon and orange. Finely grate the rind from 1 of the remaining oranges, then peel and thinly slice them both; reserve the grated rind and orange slices.

Peel the pears and place stem up, in a pan that they just fit. Add the wine, sugar, spices, bay leaves, strips of orange and lemon rind and the lemon and orange juices. Bring to the boil then cover, using a dome of foil if necessary to avoid crushing the pear stems, and simmer gently for 10 minutes. Drain the prunes and raisins, add to the pan and simmer for a further 15 minutes. Add the reserved orange slices, turn off the heat and leave the fruit to cool in the poaching liquid.

Transfer the prunes and raisins to a glass or china serving bowl and place the pears, stems up, on top. Put the orange slices round the edge.

Boil the poaching liquid over a high heat until slightly syrupy. Add the reserved grated orange rind and the ginger. Check the taste and add more ginger if needed. Discard the peppercorns, cinnamon, clove, orange and lemon rind. Leave the syrup to cool then pour, with the bay leaves, over the fruit. Serve when cold with a sweet bread or plain cake, or cover and chill.

Variation

In Burgundy a few tablespoons of *crème de cassis* are often stirred into the wine syrup just before serving (if you do this, reduce the amount of sugar you add to the pears to about 100 g/4 oz).

NUTRITIONAL INFORMATION			
One serving *Poires, Pruneaux et Oranges au Vin Rouge et aux Epices*			
Calories	318	Alcohol	20%
Fat	>1%	Vitamin A	—
Protein	3%	Vitamin C	>100%
Carbohydrate	76%	Vitamin E	2%

CLAFOUTIS

Fruit Flan

CLAUDIA RODEN

SERVES 6

Clafoutis is the perfect dessert for the French Midi with its scattered orchards and great variety of fruit. Depending on the seasons and the *pays* (regions) different fruits are dropped into a creamy batter or, as in this recipe, an egg custard, and baked in the oven.

*500 g (1 lb) cherries, plums, apricots, pears or a
mixture of 2 or more of these
4 eggs
2 egg yolks
3 tablespoons sugar*

*600 ml (1 pint) milk
4 tablespoons kirsch or cognac, or a few drops of
real vanilla essence
icing sugar*

Pre-heat the oven to gas mark 3, 160°C, 325°F. Peel the pears, cut them in half and remove the cores. Halve the plums and apricots and remove the stones. Leave cherries as they are. Spread in a buttered, shallow 30 cm (12 in) ovenproof dish.

Beat the eggs and yolks with the sugar, then beat in the milk and add the kirsch, cognac or vanilla. Pour over the fruit and bake for 45-60 minutes or until browned. Serve warm, sprinkled with icing sugar.

NUTRITIONAL INFORMATION			
One serving *Clafoutis*			
Calories	251	Protein	14%
Fat	33%	Carbohydrate	44%
of which:		Alcohol	9%
monounsaturates	43%	Vitamin A	35%
saturates	48%	Vitamin C	26%
polyunsaturates	9%	Vitamin E	18%

Sauces and Dressings

··

There is no nutritional information provided for the sauces and dressings given here as you would never be eating these quantities all at once. Instead we have added the information for a single serving of any sauce or dressing to the totals given for the main course or salad that these are served with.

Aïoli

MIREILLE JOHNSTON

SERVES 4

5 garlic cloves
2 small egg yolks
½-1 teaspoon Dijon mustard

150 ml (5 fl oz) groundnut oil
150 ml (5 fl oz) olive oil
salt and freshly ground black pepper

Crush the garlic cloves in a mortar then pound them. Stir in the egg yolks and mustard. When smooth, gradually stir in the oils a drop at a time until the sauce is smooth and quite firm. After 1 hour in the fridge it will thicken.

ROUILLE

MIREILLE JOHNSTON

SERVES 4

This fragrant sauce is based on the same principle as Mayonnaise except it is made with a pestle and mortar. If your pestle isn't big enough to take all the oil, transfer the garlic, when crushed, to a larger bowl. Keep all the ingredients at room temperature, place the mortar on a cloth and add the oil gradually.

4 garlic cloves
1 large egg yolk
120 ml (4 fl oz) olive oil
120 ml (4 fl oz) groundnut oil

juice of 1 lemon
½ teaspoon saffron strands, crushed
1 teaspoon cayenne pepper
salt and freshly ground black pepper

Crush the garlic cloves in a mortar, then pound them to a paste. Add the egg yolk, stirring and pounding constantly, then gradually stir in the oil a drop at a time. When the sauce is firm and all the oil incorporated, stir in the lemon juice, saffron, cayenne pepper, salt and pepper; the sauce should then be smooth and quite firm. After 1 hour in the fridge it will thicken.

TOMATO AND OLIVE VINAIGRETTE

DELIA SMITH

SERVES 4

225 g (8 oz) tomatoes, skinned, de-seeded and chopped small
75 g (3 oz) pitted black olives, chopped to the same size as the tomatoes
1 fat clove garlic
110 ml (4 fl oz) olive oil

1 tablespoon lemon juice
1 tablespoon white wine vinegar
1 teaspoon grain mustard
1 tablespoon chopped fresh chervil or flatleaf parsley
rock salt and freshly milled black pepper

Crush the garlic with 1 teaspoon of rock salt, using a pestle and mortar, then add the mustard, vinegar, lemon juice, olive oil and a good seasoning of black pepper, and whisk thoroughly. About half an hour before serving add the tomatoes, olives and chopped chervil or flatleaf parsley.

IL PESTO

Fresh Basil Sauce

VALENTINA HARRIS

MAKES ENOUGH TO DRESS 500 G (1¼ LB) PASTA

If you could choose one thing which says everything there is to say about Ligurian cooking, this sauce would have to be it! You can use it on any pasta shape you like, stir it into soups, pour it over boiled potatoes or use it as a dip with breadsticks. It is one of my very favourite sauces, a real Italian original, though copied by the French who have renamed it *pistou* – but they've always had problems with languages!

There are many variations on the basic sauce: some people use walnuts, others like using pine kernels; I have seen some cooks put creamy milk junket into the sauce and others who chop smoked bacon very finely and then stir that in. Like all the best recipes, it has been enjoyed enough for cooks to want to improve upon it over the decades. What is essential in any version is large amounts of fresh basil; and by this I mean at least 4 handfuls for the quantities given below, more if possible. The Genoese will tell you that the most vital point about this sauce is the instruments used to make it – you should have a marble mortar with a wooden pestle. Failing this, you will have to use a food processor.

36 leaves fresh basil, washed but not bruised,
dried carefully
large pinch rock salt
2 cloves garlic, peeled and cut in half

1 handful pine kernels
2 tablespoons grated Parmesan cheese
about ½ wine glass best-quality olive oil
salt and pepper

If you use a pestle and mortar, remember to press the basil leaves against the sides: do not bang downwards as usual. Put the basil, salt and garlic into the mortar or food processor and reduce to a smooth green purée. Add the pine kernels and cheese and blend these in also, then begin to add the oil a little at a time, until you have reached a smooth, creamy texture. Season with salt and pepper and use as required.

Basic Vinaigrette

Sophie Grigson

ENOUGH FOR A GENEROUS 6-PERSON SALAD

Please don't waste your money on bottles of ready-made French dressing. They are ridiculously expensive and not terribly good either. Making a proper vinaigrette or French dressing is child's play. Of course, you'll have to invest in a decent bottle of oil, either extra virgin olive oil or plainer groundnut oil, and another of wine vinegar, but they can be used for other things too.

Any left-over vinaigrette will keep in a screwtop jar in the fridge for several weeks. In fact, I usually make double or treble quantities, so that there's plenty left to use at a moment's notice.

1 tablespoon wine vinegar
½ teaspoon Dijon mustard (optional)

salt and freshly ground black pepper
4-5 tablespoons olive oil or groundnut oil

In a salad bowl, mix the vinegar with the mustard, salt and pepper. Whisk in the oil, a tablespoon at a time. After the fourth spoonful, taste – if it is on the sharp side, whisk in the last spoonful of oil and more if necessary. Adjust seasonings.

Alternatively put all the ingredients into a screwtop jar, close tightly and shake to mix. Taste and adjust seasoning or add more oil, as necessary.

MAYONNAISE

CLAUDIA RODEN

SERVES 4

The secret of success here lies in having all the ingredients and the bowl at room temperature and in stirring in the oil very gradually.

2 egg yolks
1½ tablespoons or more white wine vinegar or
lemon juice

salt
pinch of white pepper
300 ml (10 fl oz) olive oil

In a warm bowl, using a wooden spoon or a whisk, beat the egg yolks until they are pale, thick and sticky. Add a drop of vinegar or lemon juice and a little salt and pepper, then add the olive oil, first drop by drop, then in a thin stream, stirring vigorously all the time. As the oil becomes absorbed the sauce will thicken to a heavy, creamy consistency. If it becomes too firm, add a little more vinegar or lemon juice or a tablespoon of warm water to prevent it separating. (If the mayonnaise separates, it can be saved by starting again with a new yolk and using the sauce as if it were the oil.) I enjoy making it by hand but a blender or food processor will do the work very quickly. Simply blend the yolks with the salt, then add the oil in a thin stream while the blades are running. Add the lemon juice, then taste and adjust the seasonings.

Variations

For a green mayonnaise, add plenty of finely chopped fresh herbs, such as chives, chervil, basil, parsley, tarragon and watercress.

For a good sauce for fish, mix 3 or 4 mashed anchovies or the red eggs of sea urchins, beaten.

Italian Green Sauce

Salsa Verde

Delia Smith

SERVES 2

This is a strong-flavoured, quite garlicky sauce, which does wonders for plain mackerel fillets or some grilled trout.

4 anchovy fillets, drained
1 tablespoon capers
1 level teaspoon dry mustard powder
1 small clove garlic, crushed
1½ tablespoons lemon juice

6 tablespoons olive oil
2 tablespoons fresh chopped parsley
1 tablespoon fresh chopped basil, or
1 teaspoon dried
salt and freshly milled black pepper

To start with chop the anchovy fillets as small as possible and crush them to a paste in a mortar (if you haven't a mortar a small bowl and the end of a rolling pin will do).

Put the capers in a small sieve and rinse them under cold running water to remove the vinegar they were preserved in. Dry them on kitchen paper and chop them as minutely as you can and add them to the anchovies.

Next add the mustard, garlic, lemon juice and some freshly milled black pepper and mix well.

Now add the oil, mix again and check the taste to see how much salt to add.

Just before serving, sprinkle in the chopped herbs and again mix thoroughly so that all the ingredients are properly combined.

Note
This behaves rather like a very thick vinaigrette and, before each serving, always needs to have another mix.

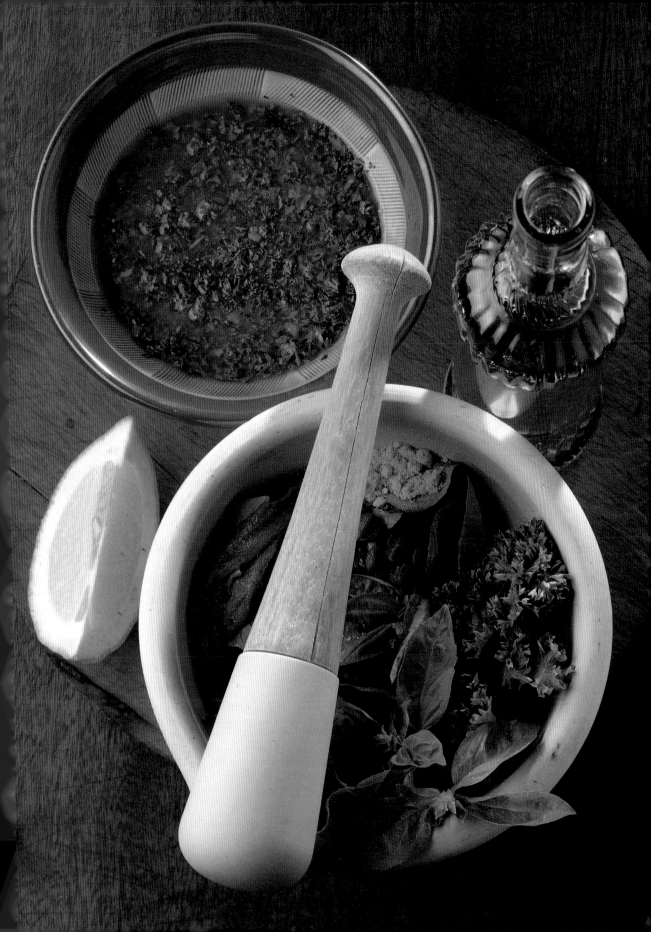

GLOSSARY

Alpha-linolenic acid (ALA) An omega 3 polyunsaturated fatty acid found in rapeseed oil.

Angina Pain from the heart caused by inadequate blood supply, usually due to atherosclerosis in the coronary arteries.

Antioxidants Chemicals which can protect against oxidation.

Atherosclerosis (or arteriosclerosis) The hardening and thickening of the artery wall which can lead to heart attacks and strokes.

Atherosclerotic plaque A large collection of fatty material in the wall of an artery.

Cholesterol level A measurement of the amount of the cholesterol in both low-density lipoprotein and high density lipoprotein.

Cis fatty acids Unsaturated fatty acids with groups of carbon atoms on the same side of the molecule (as opposed to 'trans fatty acids').

Claudication Painful cramp in the muscles of the calf or thigh during exercise.

Coronary arteries The blood vessels which supply the heart.

Coronary heart disease (coronary artery disease) Atherosclerosis and thrombosis in the coronary arteries; what happens when these blood vessels become narrowed or blocked.

Emulsifier A chemical which helps keep fats dispersed in solution.

Enzymes Chemical catalysts produced by the body.

Epidemiology The study of patterns of disease both within and between populations.

Fatty acids Organic acids which combine with glycerol to form triglycerides (fats).

Flavonoids Types of naturally occurring antioxidant chemical which occur in a wide variety of fruit and vegetables.

Folic acid A vitamin of the B group which is present in all green plants.

Foam cells Frothy-looking cells filled with cholesterol and other fats.

Free radical An especially reactive atom which is unstable and reacts readily with other molecules – often produced by 'oxidation'.

Gangrene The death of the tissues of the toes or feet.

Glycerol The chemical forming the backbone of fats and oils – triglycerides.

Hardening of the arteries A term used to mean atherosclerosis.

Heart failure The accumulation of fluid in the lungs or the legs resulting from weakness of the heart's pumping function.

High-density lipoprotein Lipid particles which protect against vascular disease, also known as 'good' cholesterol.

Hydrogenation The process of adding hydrogen to a substance, especially a fatty acid; used to 'harden' vegetable oils to make some margarines.

Low-density lipoprotein Lipid particles which help cause vascular disease; the main form of 'bad' cholesterol.

Monounsaturated fatty acid Fatty acid containing one unsaturated (double) chemical bond.

Myocardial infarction A heart attack, where heart muscle dies because of loss of blood supply.

Omega 3 fatty acids An unsaturated fatty acid with its first double, unsaturated, bond three carbons up from the far end; found in fish and rapeseed oil.

Omega 6 fatty acids An unsaturated fatty acid with its first double, unsaturated, bond six carbons up from the far end; found in most vegetable oils.

Oxidation Process of damage, which can happen to several chemicals in the body, in which they are attacked by a supercharged form of oxygen. When this happens to fats, they go rancid.

Ozone A supercharged form of oxygen.

Platelets The cells in the blood which start the clotting process.

Polyunsaturated fatty acids Fatty acids containing more than one unsaturated (double) chemical bond.

Risk factors Physical, chemical, behavioural or environmental characteristics which increase the likelihood of developing a disease.

Salicylic acid Aspirin.

Saturated fatty acids Fatty acids in which all the carbon atoms are joined by single bonds. These fats are chiefly of animal origin.

Stroke Produced by a blood clot in an artery supplying the brain, usually causing paralysis of part of the body.

Thrombosis Blood clotting which, if it happens in an artery, can directly cause a heart attack or stroke. This usually happens where an artery is affected by atherosclerosis.

Thrombus Blood clot.

Trans fatty acids Unsaturated fatty acids with groups of carbon atoms on opposite sides of the molecule (as opposed to 'Cis fatty acids').

Triglyceride The sort of fat in animal fat or vegetable oil made up of glycerol and three fatty acids.

Unsaturated fatty acids Fatty acids containing at least one unsaturated, double, bond between the carbon atoms. These bonds are easily split in chemical reactions and other substances joined to them.

BIBLIOGRAPHY

Chapter 1

Page 12:   Data from: British Heart Foundation, *Statistical Report* (1993).

Page 13:   Copied from: British Heart Foundation, (1993).

Page 14:   Adapted from: various including Multiple Risk Factor Intervention Trial Research Group JAMA (1982), 248: 1465-77 and Kannel, W.B. et al., (1971), *Annals of Internal Medicine*, 74: 1-12.

Page 16:   Data from: Yudkin, J.S., *British Medical Journal* (1993), 306: 1313-1318

Page 18:   Copied from: Keys, A., et al., *Circulation* (1970), Suppl. XLI-XLII.

Chapter 2

Page 19:   Data from: British Heart Foundation *Statistical Report* (1993).

Page 22:   Data from: Renaud, S. and de Lorgeril, M., *The Lancet* (1992), 339: 1523-26.

Page 24:   Data from: Criqui, M.H., et al., *The Lancet* (1994), 344: 1719-23.

Chapter 3

Page 31:   Copied from: Keys, A., et al., *Circulation* (1970), Suppl. XLI-XLII.

Page 32:   Copied from: Renaud, S. and de Lorgeril, M., *The Lancet* (1992), 339: 1523-26.

Page 33:   Data from: Shekelle, R.B., *New England Journal of Medicine* (1981), 304: 65-70.

Page 36:   Data from: Mensink, R.P., and Katan, M.B., *New England Journal of Medicine* (1990), 323: 439-45.

Page 39:   Adapted from: McCance, R.A., and Widdowson, E.M., *The Composition of Foods* (1991), Cambridge, Royal Society of Chemistry.

Page 40:   Data from: Ginsberg, H.N. et al., *New England Journal of Medicine* (1990), 322: 574-9.

Page 43:   Data from: *Balance and Lifestyle* British Diabetic Association (Feb/Mar 1995).

Chapter 4

Page 51:   Copied from: Criqui, M.H., et al., *The Lancet* (1994), 344: 1719-23.

Chapter 5

Page 54:   Data from: Criqui, M.H., et al., *The Lancet* (1994), 344: 1719-23.

Page 55:   Copied from Criqui, M.H., et al., *The Lancet* (1994), 344: 1719-23.

Page 57:   Copied from Criqui, M.H., et al., *The Lancet* (1994), 344: 1719-23.

Page 58:   Copied from: Renaud, S. and de Lorgeril, M., *The Lancet* (1992), 339: 1523-6.

Chapter 6

Page 66:   Data from: Kromhout, D., et al., *New England Journal of Medicine* (1985), 312: 1205-9.

Page 67:   Burr, M.L., et al., *The Lancet* (1989), 33: 757-761.

Chapter 7

Page 71:   COMA Report copied from:MAFF: *Household Food Consumption and Expenditure 1990, 1991, 1992, (1991, 1992, 1993)*, London, HMSO.

Page 72:   Excerpted with permission from: Willett, W.C., *Science* (1994), 264: 532-7.

Page 72   Data from: the Seven Countries Study, Keys, A., et al., *Circulation* (1970), Suppl. XLI-XLII.

Chapter 8

Page 78:   Data from Yudkin, J.S., *British Medical Journal* (1993), 306:1313-1318

The authors have made every effort to trace copyright holders of material used in this book. If, however, they have inadvertently made any error they would be grateful for notification.

INDEX